ATLAS OF
INFECTIOUS DISEASES OF THE
FEMALE GENITAL TRACT

ATLAS OF INFECTIOUS DISEASES OF THE FEMALE GENITAL TRACT

RICHARD L. SWEET, MD

Professor
Department of Obstetrics and Gynecology
University of California, Davis
Director, Center for Women's Health
University of California Davis Medical Center

RONALD S. GIBBS, MD

E. Stewart Taylor Chair in Obstetrics and Gynecology
Professor and Chair
Department of Obstetrics and Gynecology
University of Colorado Health Sciences Center
Denver, Colorado

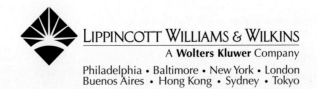

LIPPINCOTT WILLIAMS & WILKINS
A **Wolters Kluwer** Company

Philadelphia • Baltimore • New York • London
Buenos Aires • Hong Kong • Sydney • Tokyo

Acquisitions Editor: Ruth Weinberg
Developmental Editor: Nicole T. Dernoski
Project Manager: Nicole Walz
Senior Manufacturing Manager: Benjamin Rivera
Production Editor: Barbara Stabb, TechBooks
Cover Designer: Melissa Walter
Design Coordinator: Holly McLaughlin
Compositor: TechBooks
Printer: Quebecor World-Kingsport

Library of Congress Cataloging-in-Publication Data
Sweet, Richard L.
   Atlas of infectious diseases of the female genital tract / Richard L. Sweet, Ronald S. Gibbs.
      p. ; cm.
   Includes index.
   Companion v. to: Infectious diseases of the female genital tract. 4th ed. c2002.
   ISBN 0-7817-5583-2 (alk. paper)
   1. Generative organs, Female—Infections—Atlases.   2. Generative organs, Female—Microbiology—Atlases.   I. Gibbs, Ronald S., 1943-   II. Sweet, Richard L. Infectious diseases of the female genital tract.   III. Title.
   [DNLM: 1. Genital Diseases, Female—Atlases.   2. Communicable Diseases—Atlases. 3. Pregnancy Complications, Infectious—Atlases.   WP 17 S974a 2004]
RG79. S93 2004
618.1—dc22
                                                                              2004016167

We dedicate this atlas to our wives, Rhea and Jane, for their continued love, support, and understanding. To our children, Jennifer and Troy, Suzanne and Darragh, Andrew and Inga, Eric and Whitney, Stuart and Suzanne, and our grandchildren Hanna, Dylan, Emily, Benjamin, Paige, Samantha, Jordan, Tanner, and future grandchildren who inspire us to continue our commitment to education and teaching of infectious diseases as they relate to women's health.

PREFACE

We are delighted to see the publication of this atlas to accompany our text, *Infectious Diseases of the Female Genital Tract*, now in its fourth edition. The purpose of the atlas is to provide a clinically useful source including photographs to illustrate disease processes and facilitate diagnoses. In addition, we have included a number of graphs and tables to summarize diagnoses and treatment.

Public attention has continued to focus on infectious diseases in the last few years with developments in HIV, severe acute respiratory syndrome (SARS), anthrax, and West Nile virus. Infectious diseases continue to play an important role in the practice of obstetrics and gynecology, and infection/inflammation appear to have a broadening role in processes as diverse as genital cancer and preterm birth. We hope that this new volume will earn a place in the offices and libraries of many physicians. We are grateful for their continuing interest in our texts.

CONTENTS

INTRODUCTION

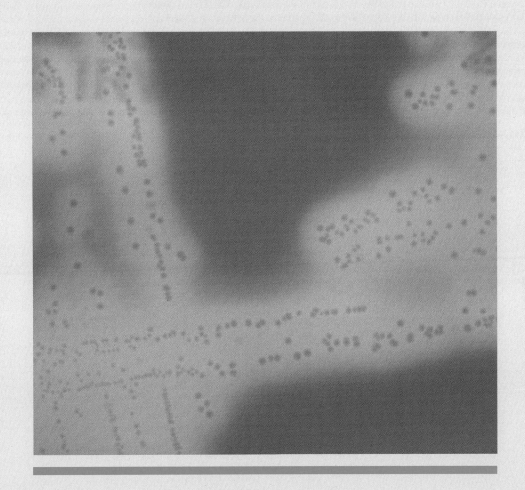

1

CLINICAL MICROBIOLOGY AND USE OF THE MICROBIOLOGY LAB IN INFECTIOUS DISEASES OF THE FEMALE GENITAL TRACT

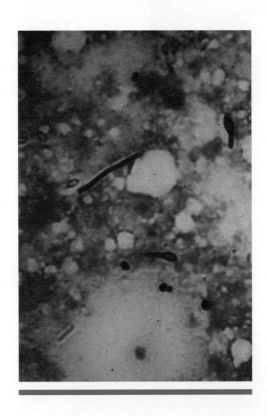

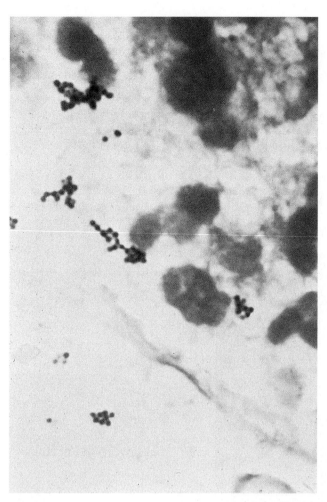

FIGURE 1.1 Gram stain of the *Staphylococcus aureus* in a clinical specimen.

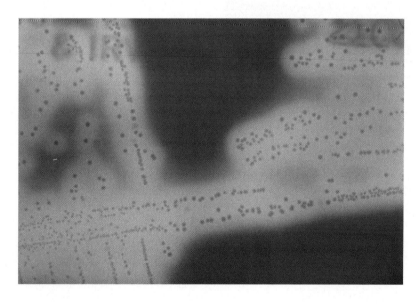

FIGURE 1.2 Close-up view of colonies of Group A Streptococci on a blood agar plate. Note the zone of clear hemolysis.

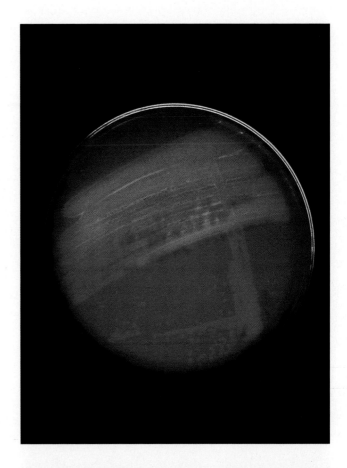

FIGURE 1.3 A blood agar plate showing partial (alpha) or green hemolysis. This is characteristic of the alpha hemolytic streptococci.

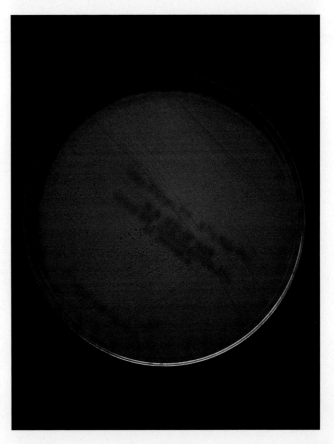

FIGURE 1.4 A blood agar plate showing nonhemolytic colonies of enterococci.

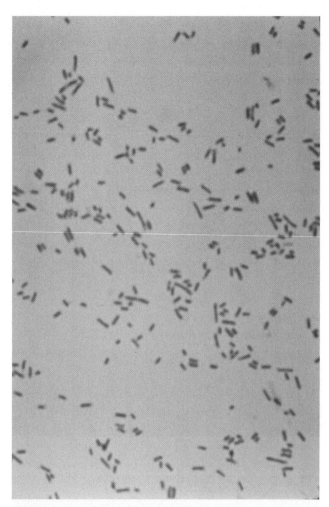

FIGURE 1.5 Gram stain showing gram-negative rods picked from a colony on an agar plate.

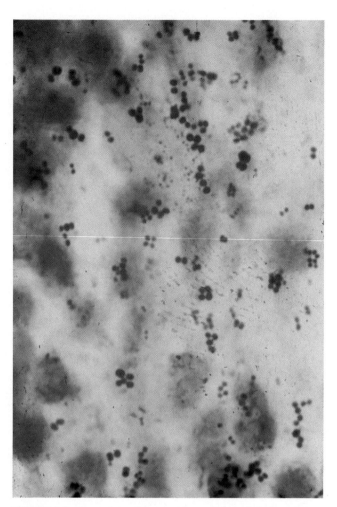

FIGURE 1.6 Gram stain of anaerobic cocci in a clinical specimen.

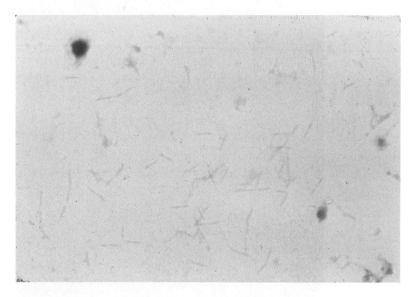

FIGURE 1.7 Gram stain showing *Bacteroides fragilis*.

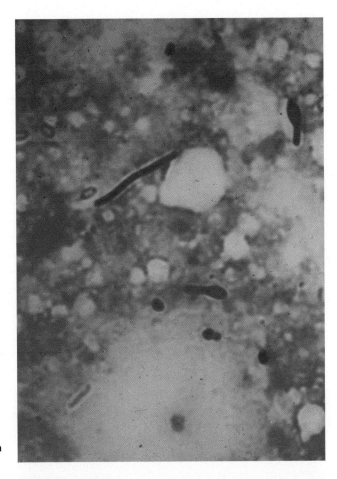

FIGURE 1.8 Gram stain showing *Clostridium perfringens* from a clinical specimen.

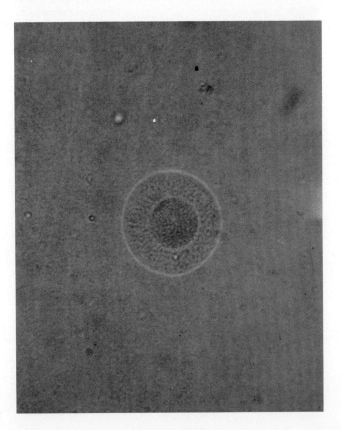

FIGURE 1.9 A colony of *Mycoplasma hominis* in culture.

TABLE 1.1 ANTIBIOTIC THERAPY FOR AEROBIC AND FACULTATIVE BACTERIA FOUND IN FEMALE GENITAL INFECTIONS

Aerobic and Facultative Bacteria	Recommended Antibiotic(s)	Alternative Antibiotic(s)
Gram-positive cocci		
Staphylococcus aureus	Penicillinase-resistant penicillin	Vancomycin, cephalosporin
Staphylococcus epidermidis[a]	Rarely causes pelvic infection	
Staphylococcus saprophyticus	Penicillin, TMP-SMX	Cephalosporin
Enterococcus faecalis (group D enterococcus)	Ampicillin, ampicillin + gentamicin	Vancomycin
Streptococcus agalactiae (group B streptococcus)	Penicillin, ampicillin	Clindamycin, cephalosporin
Streptococcus pneumoniae (Diplococcus pneumoniae)	Penicillin	Clindamycin, vancomycin, clarithromycin
Streptococcus pyogenes (group A streptococcus)	Penicillin	Erythromycin, cephalosporin, clindamycin, vancomycin
Viridans group streptococci	Penicillin and gentamicin	Cephalosporin, vancomycin
Gram-positive bacilli		
Corynebacterium sp[a]	Rarely cause pelvic infection	
Gardnerella vaginalis[b]	Mainly treated as part of bacterial vaginosis flora	
Diphtheroids[a]	Rarely causes pelvic infection	
Lactobacillus sp[a]	Rarely causes pelvic infection	
Listeria monocytogenes	Ampicillin (± gentamicin)	Cephalosporin, TMP-SMX
Gram-negative cocci		
Neisseria gonorrhoeae	Cefixime, ceftriaxone, ciprofloxacin, or ofloxacin	Spectinomycin, other single-dose cephalosporins, or quinolones
Gram-negative bacilli		
Enterobacter sp	Newer cephalosporins	Aminoglycoside, TMP-SMX
Escherichia coli	For sepsis, gentamicin ± cephalosporin or extended spectrum penicillin. For urinary tract infection, TMP-SMX, TMP	Some newer cephalosporins, TMP-SMX
Klebsiella pneumoniae	Newer cephalosporins, gentamicin	TMP-SMX
Proteus mirabilis	Ampicillin, amoxicillin	Cephalosporins, gentamicin, TMP-SMX, quinolones
Pseudomonas aeruginosa	Aminoglycoside + ticarcillin	Newer cephalosporins ± aminoglycoside

[a]Species generally with low virulence.
[b]G. vaginalis may be a coccobacillus.
SMX, sulfamethoxazole; TMP, trimethoprim.

TABLE 1.2 ANTIBIOTIC THERAPY FOR ANAEROBIC BACTERIA FOUND IN FEMALE GENITAL INFECTION

Anaerobic Bacteria	Recommended Antibiotic(s)	Alternative Antibiotic(s)
Gram-positive cocci		
Peptostreptococcus	Penicillin, clindamycin, matronidazole	Cefoxitin, selected other cephalosporins
Peptostreptococcus anaerobius		
Peptostreptococcus asaccharolyticus		
Peptostreptococcus magnus		
Peptostreptococcus prevotii		
Gram-positive bacilli		
Actinomyces sp	Penicillins	Most cephalosporins, tetracycline, rifampin
Propionibacterium sp[a]	Rarely cause pelvic infection	
Clostridium perfringens	Penicillin, clindamycin, cefoxitin	Chloramphenicol, imipenem
Clostridium sp	Usually penicillin, metronidazole, clindamycin	
Clostridium difficile	Metronidazole, vancomycin	
Gram-negative bacilli		
Bacteroides (*Bacteroides fragilis* group)	Metronidazole, selected penicillin β-lactamase inhibitors, imipenem	Cefoxitin, cefotetan, clindamycin
Bacteroides sp, other	Clindamycin, metronidaxole, cefoxitin, penicillin β-inhibitors, cefotetan	Selected other cephalosporins
Fusobacterium sp		
Porphyromonas asaccharolytica		
Prevotella bivia		
Prevotella disiens		
Prevotella melaninogenica		

[a]Species generally with low virulence.

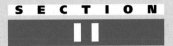

SPECIAL ORGANISMS

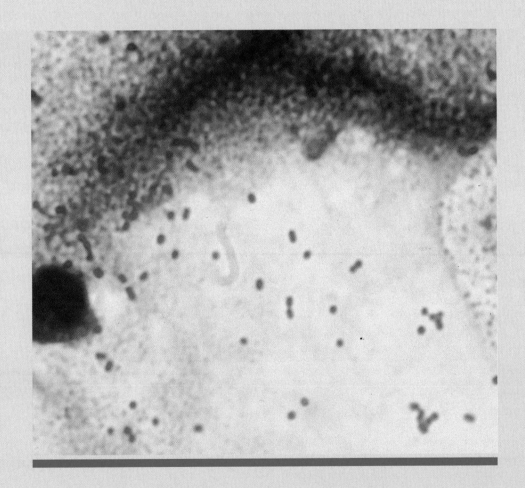

2

GROUP B STREPTOCOCCI

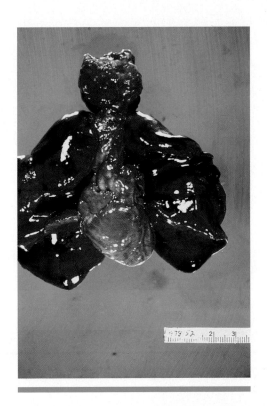

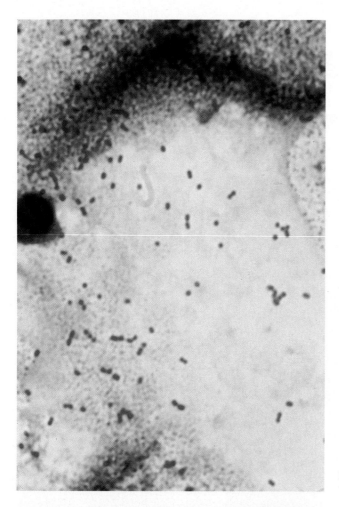

FIGURE 2.1 Gram stain of Group B Streptococci in the amniotic fluid of a patient with chorioamnionitis.

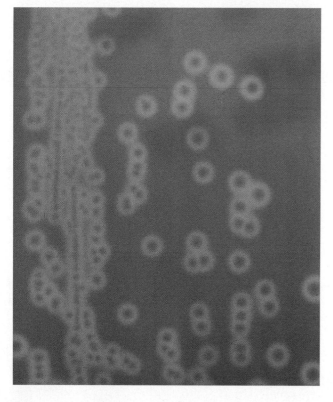

FIGURE 2.2 Colonies of Group B Streptococci on a blood agar plate. Note the zone of clear hemolysis.

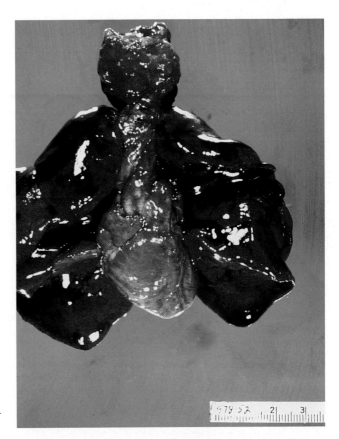

FIGURE 2.3 A heart/lung dissection of an infant who died of overwhelming Group B Streptococcal sepsis and pneumonia.

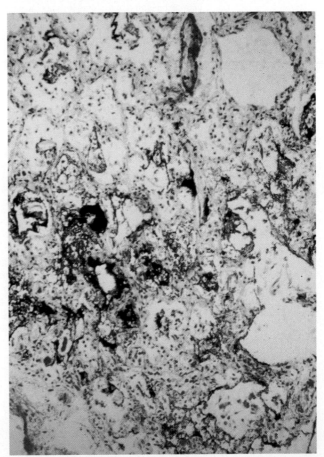

FIGURE 2.4 Gram stain of the lungs of an infant with overwhelming Group B Streptococci. Note the extensive number of gram positive cocci in tissues.

Vaginal and rectal GBS screening cultures at 35–37 weeks' gestation for **ALL** pregnant women (unless patient had GBS bacteriuria during the current pregnancy or a previous infant with invasive GBS disease)

Intrapartum prophylaxis indicated

- Previous infant with invasive GBS disease

- GBS bacteriuria during current pregnancy

- Positive GBS screening culture during current pregnancy (unless a planned cesarean delivery, in the absence of labor or amniotic membrane rupture, is performed)

- Unknown GBS status (culture not done, incomplete, or results unknown) and any of the following:
    - Delivery at <37 weeks' gestation[a]
    - Amniotic membrane rupture ≥18 hours
    - Intrapartum temperature ≥ 100.4°F (≥38.0°C)[b]

Intrapartum prophylaxis not indicated

- Previous pregnancy with a positive GBS screening culture (unless a culture was also positive during the current pregnancy)

- Planned cesarean delivery performed in the absence of labor or membrane rupture (regardless of maternal GBS culture status)

- Negative vaginal and rectal GBS screening culture in late gestation during the current pregnancy, regardless of intrapartum risk factors

[a]If onset of labor or rupture of amniotic membranes occurs at <37 weeks' gestation and there is a significant risk for preterm delivery (as assessed by the clinician), a suggested algorithm for GBS prophylaxis management is provided (Fig. 2.6).

[b]If amnionitis is suspected, broad-spectrum antibiotic therapy that includes an agent known to be active against GBS should replace GBS prophylaxis.

FIGURE 2.5 Indications for intrapartum antibiotic prophylaxis to prevent perinatal GBS disease under a universal prenatal screening strategy based on combined vaginal and rectal cultures collected at 35–37 weeks' gestation from all pregnant women. (From Centers for Disease Control and Prevention. Prevention of Perinatal Group B Streptococcal Disease. *MMWR* 2002;51[No. RR-11]:8, with permission.)

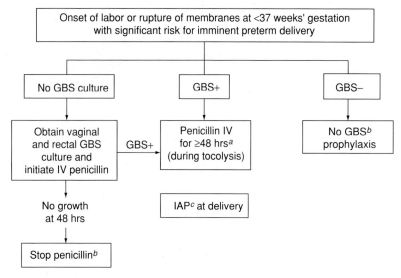

[a]Penicillin should be continued for a total of at least 48 hours, unless delivery occurs sooner. At the physician's discretion, antibiotic prophylaxis may be continued beyond 48 hours in a GBS culture-positive woman if delivery has not yet occurred. For women who are GBS culture positive, antibiotic prophylaxis should be reinitiated when labor likely to proceed to delivery occurs or recurs.

[b]If delivery has not occurred within 4 weeks, a vaginal and rectal GBS screening culture should be repeated and the patient should be managed as described, based on the result of the repeat culture.

[c]Intrapartum antibiotic prophylaxis.

FIGURE 2.6 Sample algorithm for GBS prophylaxis for women with threatened preterm delivery. This algorithm is not an exclusive course of management. Variations that incorporate individual circumstances or institutional preferences may be appropriate. (From Centers for Disease Control and Prevention. Prevention of Perinatal Group B Streptococcal Disease. *MMWR* 2002;51[No. RR-11]:12, with permission.)

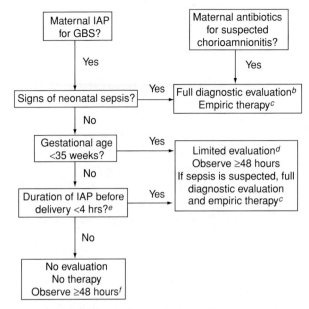

a If no maternal intrapartum prophylaxis for GBS was administered despite an indication being present, data are insufficient on whether to recommend a single management strategy.

b Includes complete blood cell count and differential, blood culture, and chest radiograph if respiratory abnormalities are present. When signs of sepsis are present, a lumbar puncture, if feasible, should be performed.

c Duration of therapy varies depending on results of blood culture, cerebrospinal fluid findings, if obtained, and the clinical course of the infant. If laboratory results and clinical course do not indicate bacterial infection, duration may be as short as 48 hours.

d CBC with differential and blood culture.

e Applies only to penicillin, ampicillin, or cefazolin and assumes recommended dosing regimens (Box 2.1).

f A healthy-appearing infant who was ≥38 weeks' gestation at delivery and whose mother received ≥4 hours of intrapartum prophylaxis before delivery may be discharged home after 24 hours if other discharge criteria have been met and a person able to comply fully with instructions for home observation will be present. If any one of these conditions is not met, the infant should be observed in the hospital for at least 48 hours and until criteria for discharge are achieved.

FIGURE 2.7 Sample algorithm for management of a newborn whose mother received intrapartum antimicrobial agents for prevention of early-onset group B streptococcal disease[a] or suspected chorioamnionitis. This algorithm is not an exclusive course of management. Variations that incorporate individual circumstances or institutional preferences may be appropriate. (From Centers for Disease Control and Prevention. *Prevention of Perinatal Group B Streptococcal Disease. MMWR* 2002;51[No. RR-11]:13, with permission.)

BOX 2.1
Recommended Regimens for Intrapartum Antimicrobial Prophylaxis for Perinatal GBS Disease Prevention[a]

Recommended Regimen
- Penicillin G 5 million units IV initial dose, then 2.5 million units IV every 4 hours until delivery

Alternative Regimen
- Ampicillin 2 g IV initial dose, then 1 g IV every 4 hours until delivery

If Penicillin Allergic[b]

Patients not at high risk for anaphylaxis
- Cefazolin 2 g IV initial dose, then 1 g IV every 8 hours until delivery

Patients at high risk for anaphylaxis[c]: GBS susceptible to clindamycin and erythromycin[d]
- Clindamycin 900 mg IV every 8 hours until delivery
  or
- Erythromycin 500 mg IV every 6 hours until delivery

Patients at high risk for anaphylaxis: GBS resistant to clindamycin or erythromycin or susceptibility unknown
- Vancomycin[e] 1 g IV every 12 hours until delivery

---

[a] Broader-spectrum agents, including an agent active against GBS, may be necessary for treatment of chorioamnionitis.

[b] History of penicillin allergy should be assessed to determine whether a high risk for anaphylaxis is present. Penicillin-allergic patients at high risk for anaphylaxis are those who have experienced immediate hypersensitivity to penicillin including a history of penicillin-related anaphylaxis; other high-risk patients are those with asthma or other diseases that would make anaphylaxis more dangerous or difficult to treat, such as persons being treated with beta-adrenergic-blocking agents.

[c] If laboratory facilities are adequate, clindamycin and erythromycin susceptibility testing should be performed on prenatal GBS isolates from penicillin-allergic women at high risk for anaphylaxis.

[d] Resistance to erythromycin is often but not always associated with clindamycin resistance. If a strain is resistant to erythromycin but appears susceptible to clindamycin, it may still have inducible resistance to clindamycin.

[e] Cefazolin is preferred over vancomycin for women with a history of penicillin allergy other than immediate hypersensitivity reactions, and pharmacologic data suggest it achieves effective intraamniotic concentrations. Vancomycin should be reserved for penicillin-allergic women at high risk for anaphylaxis.

Note: From Centers for Disease Control and Prevention. Prevention of Perinatal Group B Streptococcal Disease. *MMWR* 2002;51(No. RR-11):10, with permission.

3

GENITAL MYCOPLASMAS

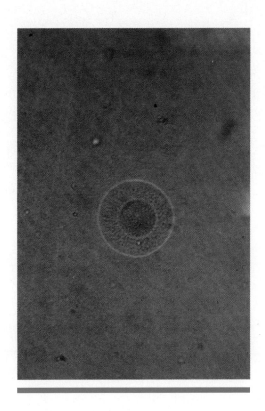

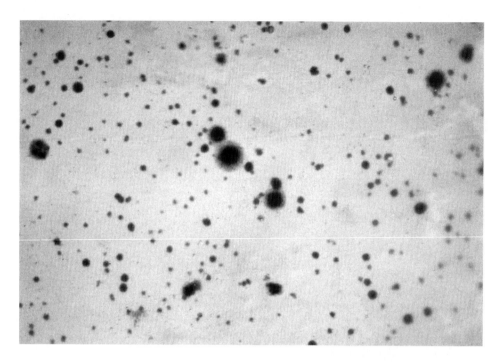

FIGURE 3.1 *Mycoplasma hominis* and *Ureaplasma urealyticum* on a selective agar plate. *Mycoplasma hominis* appears as the larger "fried egg" colonies.

4

CHLAMYDIAL INFECTIONS

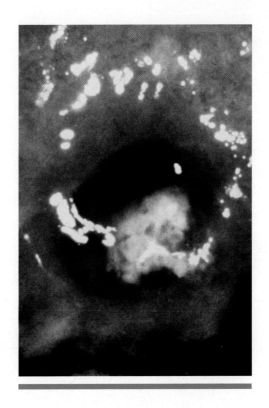

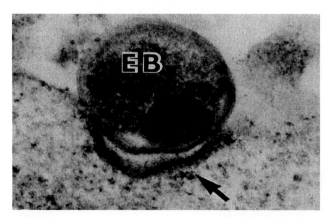

FIGURE 4.1 Elementary body, the infectious form, of *Chlamydia trachomatis*.

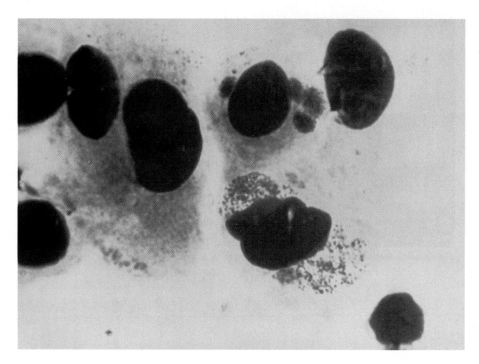

FIGURE 4.2 Giemsa stain demonstrating *Chlamydia trachomatis* inclusions.

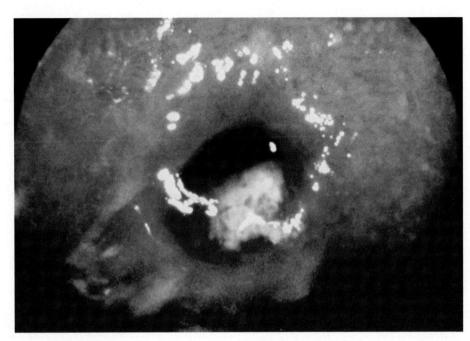

FIGURE 4.3 *Chlamydial mucopurulent cervicitis.*

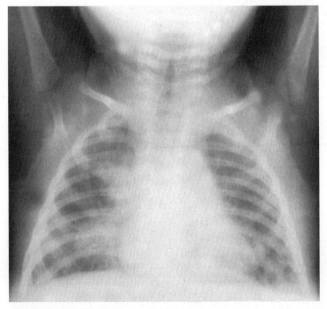

FIGURE 4.4 *Chlamydial pneumonia* of newborn.

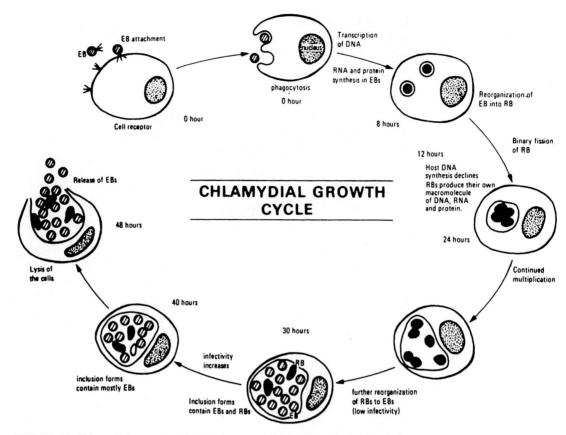

FIGURE 4.5 Chlamydial growth cycle. EB, elementary body; RB, reticulate body. (From Thompson SE, Washington AE. Epidemiology of sexually transmitted *Chlamydia trachomatis* infections. *Epidemiol Rev* 1983;5:96–123, with permission.)

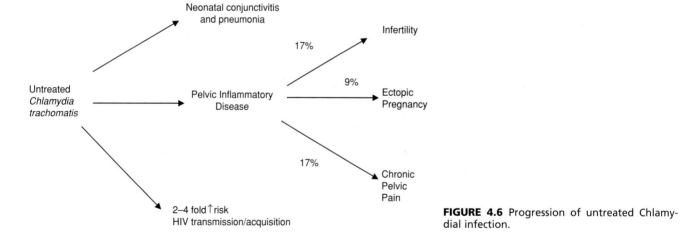

FIGURE 4.6 Progression of untreated Chlamydial infection.

BOX 4.1

Recommended Regimens for Chlamydial Infection of the Lower Genital Tract

Recommended Regimen
- Azithromycin 1 g PO in a single dose
  or
- Doxycycline 100 mg PO b.i.d. for 7 days

Alternative Regimen
- Erythromycin base 500 mg PO q.i.d. for 7 days
  or
- Ofloxacin 300 mg PO b.i.d. for 7 days
  or
- Levofloxacin 500 mg PO daily for 7 days

Note: From Centers for Disease Control and Prevention. Sexually transmitted diseases treatment guidelines. *MMWR* 2002;51(RR-6):1–78, with permission.

BOX 4.2

Recommended Regimens for Chlamydial Genital Tract Infections During Pregnancy

Recommended Regimen
- Erythromycin base 500 mg PO q.i.d. for 7 days
  or
- Amoxicillin 500 mg PO t.i.d. for 7 days

Alternative Regimen
- Erythromycin base 250 mg PO q.i.d. for 14 days
  or
- Erythromycin ethylsuccinate 800 mg PO q.i.d. for 7 days
  or
- Erythromycin ethylsuccinate 400 mg PO q.i.d. for 14 days
  or
- Azithromycin 1 g PO in a single dose

Note: From Centers for Disease Control and Prevention. Sexually transmitted diseases treatment guidelines. *MMWR* 2002;51(RR-6):1–78, with permission.

5

HERPES SIMPLEX VIRUS INFECTION

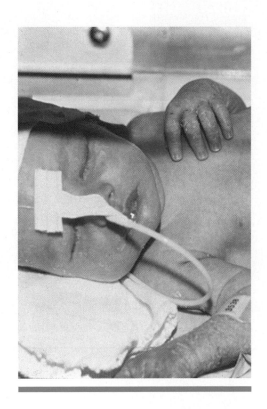

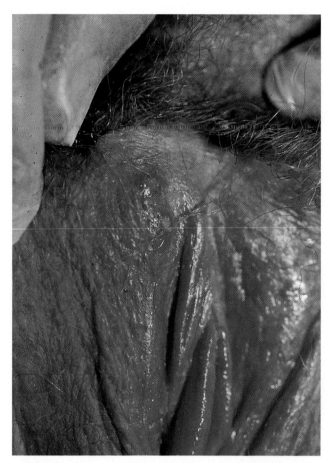

FIGURE 5.1 Herpetic vesicles on the labia in a patient at 14 weeks' gestation.

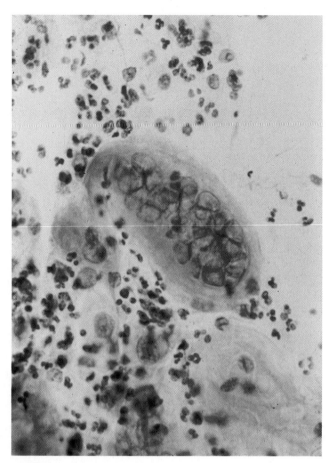

FIGURE 5.2 Papanicolaou smear showing multinucleated giant cells characteristic of herpes simplex infection.

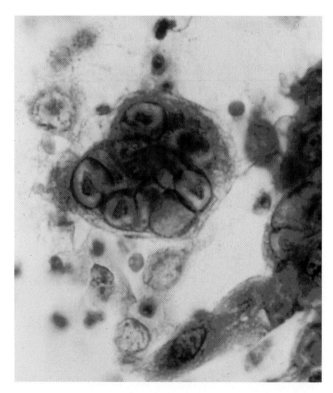

FIGURE 5.3 Papanicolaou smear showing multinucleated giant cells with intranuclear inclusions from a case of herpes simplex infection.

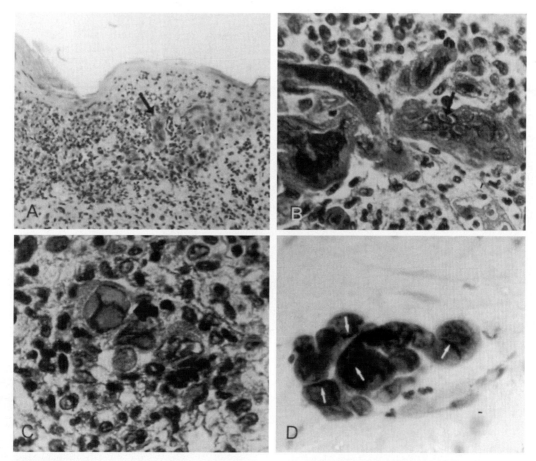

FIGURE 5.4 Characteristic histologic changes seen in herpes simplex virus infection of the vulva. **A:** Necrosis of the epidermis and dermis, with acute inflammation and nuclear debris (*left*), viable mucosal keratinocytes (*right*), and multinucleated giant cells (*center; arrow*) (hematoxylin-eosin, original magnification ×90). **B:** Multinucleated cells with Cowdry type A intranuclear viral inclusions (*arrow*) (hematoxylin-eosin, original magnification ×220). **C:** Nuclear molding (the contours of adjacent nuclei conform to one another) with a ground-glass chromatin pattern (*arrow*) in an enlarged, multinucleated cell (hematoxylin-eosin, original magnification ×480). **D:** Vaginal smear shows margination by nuclear chromatin (*arrows*) (Papanicolaou stain, original magnification ×550). (From Brennick J, Duncan L. Images in clinical medicine. *N Engl Med* 1994;329:1783, with permission.)

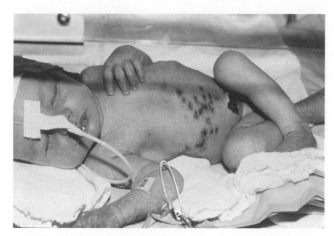

FIGURE 5.5 Newborn with disseminated herpes simplex virus infection. Note the healing ulcerations on the abdomen of the infant.

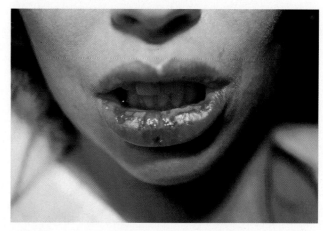

FIGURE 5.6 Herpes labialis due to herpes simplex virus type I in a pregnant woman.

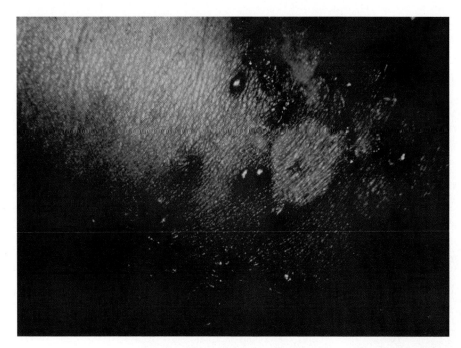

FIGURE 5.7 Cutaneous congenital Herpes simplex infection in newborn.

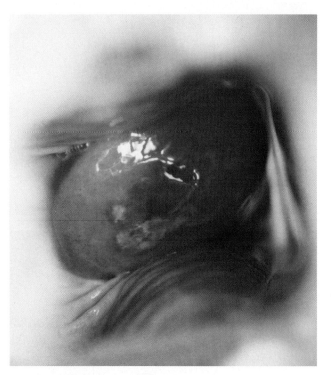

FIGURE 5.8 Herpes cervicitis.

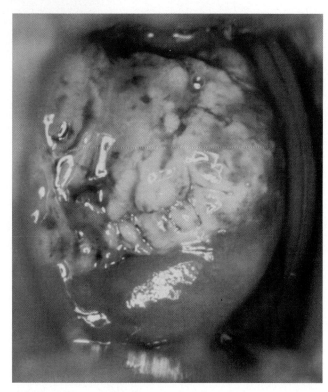

FIGURE 5.9 Herpes simplex cervicitis.

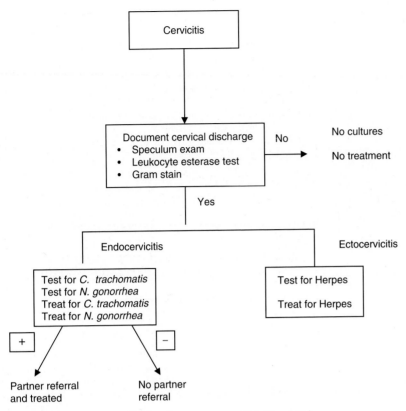

FIGURE 5.10 Follow up if symptoms recur or persist. (Cervicitis)

BOX 5.1
Recommended Regimens for Genital Herpes

Recommended Regimen for first Clinical Episode of Genital Herpes[a]
- Acyclovir 400 mg PO t.i.d. for 7–10 days
  or
- Acyclovir 200 mg PO five times a day for 7–10 days
  or
- Famciclovir 250 mg PO t.i.d. for 7–10 days
  or
- Valacyclovir 1 g PO b.i.d. for 7–10 days

Recommended Regimen for Episodic Recurrent Infection
- Acyclovir 400 mg PO t.i.d. for 5 days
  or
- Acyclovir 200 mg PO five times a day for 5 days
  or
- Acyclovir 800 mg PO b.i.d. for 5 days
  or
- Famciclovir 125 mg PO b.i.d. for 5 days
  or
- Valacyclovir 500 mg PO b.i.d. for 5 days
  or
- Valacyclovir 1 g PO q.d. for 5 days

Recommended Regimen for Daily Suppressive Therapy
- Acyclovir 400 mg PO b.i.d.
  or
- Famciclovir 250 mg PO b.i.d.
  or
- Valacyclovir 250 mg PO b.i.d.
  or
- Valacyclovir 500 mg PO q.d.
  or
- Valacyclovir 1,000 mg PO q.d.

---

[a]Treatment may be extended if healing is incomplete after 10 days of therapy.
Note: From Centers for Disease Control and Prevention. Sexually transmitted diseases treatment guidelines. *MMWR* 2002;51 (RR-6):14–16, with permission.

BOX 5.2
Management of Genital Herpes Simplex Virus in Pregnancy: Recurrent Infection

- Counsel, educate, reassure
- Do not perform routine cultures
- Examine on admission to labor and delivery unit
- Anticipate vaginal delivery
- Acyclovir prophylaxis is not established

BOX 5.3
Management of Genital Herpes Simplex Virus in Pregnancy: First-Episode Infection

- Consultation may be appropriate
- Establish HSV infection as primary, nonprimary, or recurrent, if possible
- Educate and evaluate for intrauterine growth retardation, intrauterine fetal death, preterm labor, and neonatal infection, when appropriate
- Acyclovir prophylaxis to prevent maternal recurrences is not established

BOX 5.4
Management of Genital Herpes Simplex Virus in Pregnancy: In Labor

- If there is a lesion or a typical prodrome, perform a cesarean delivery, ideally before membrane rupture
- If there is no infection, allow vaginal delivery
- Inform nursery about maternal history

6

SEXUALLY TRANSMITTED DISEASES

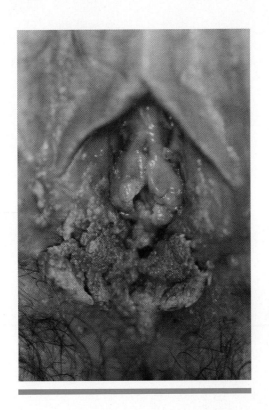

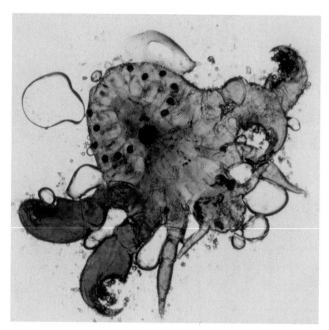

FIGURE 6.1 *Pthirius pubis,* the crab louse. Etiologic agent Pediculosis pubis.

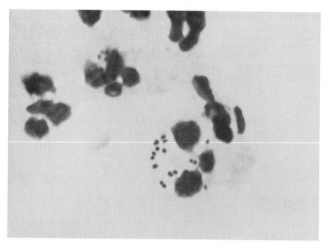

FIGURE 6.2 Gram negative intracellular diplococci of *N. gonorrhoeae* on Gram stain.

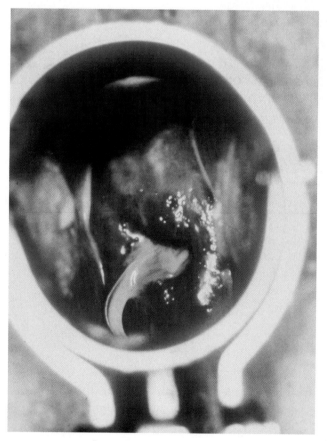

FIGURE 6.3 Gonococcal mucopurulent cervicitis.

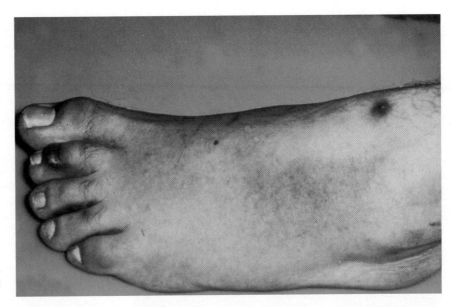

FIGURE 6.4 Disseminated gonorrhea: pustule with hemorrhagic base and necrotic center.

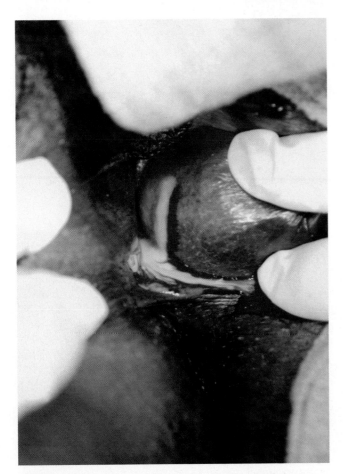

FIGURE 6.5 Purulent drainage from Bartholin gland abscess.

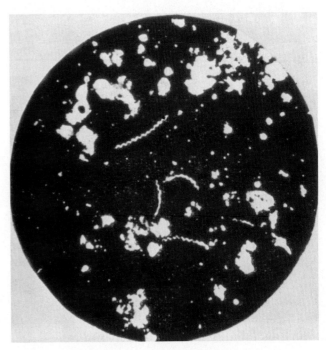

FIGURE 6.6 Silver stain of Treponema pallidum spirochete.

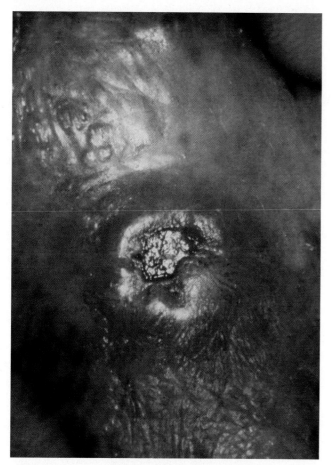

FIGURE 6.7 Chancre of primary syphilis.

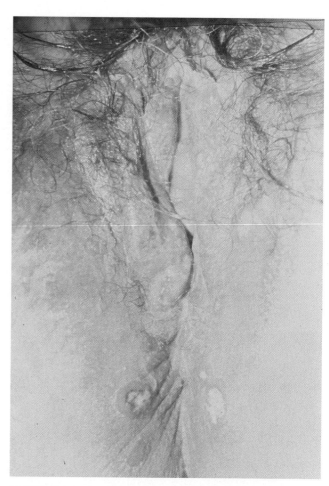

FIGURE 6.9 Perineal chancre in a case of primary syphilis.

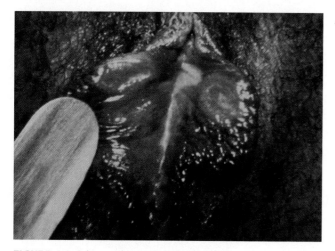

FIGURE 6.8 Primary chancre of syphilis on labia.

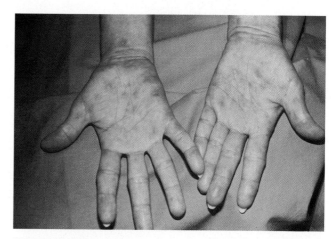

FIGURE 6.10 Maculopapular rash on the palms characteristic of secondary syphilis.

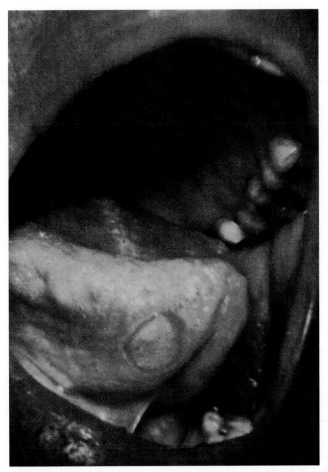

FIGURE 6.11 Mucous patch of tongue in secondary syphilis.

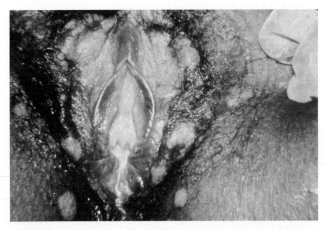

FIGURE 6.13 Sessile genital warts of condyloma lata, a manifestation of secondary syphilis.

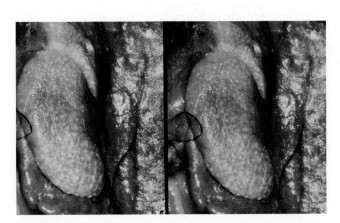

FIGURE 6.12 Condyloma latum of secondary syphilis.

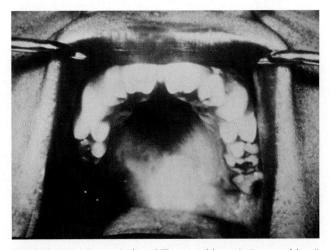

FIGURE 6.14 Congenital syphilis—Hutchinson's "screw driver" incisors.

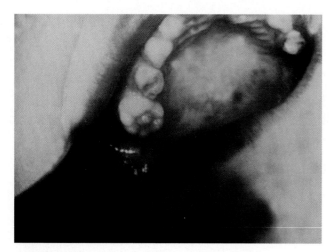

FIGURE 6.15 Congenital syphilis—mulberry molar.

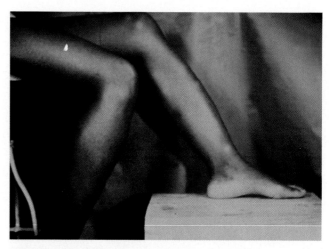

FIGURE 6.16 Saber shins of congenital syphilis.

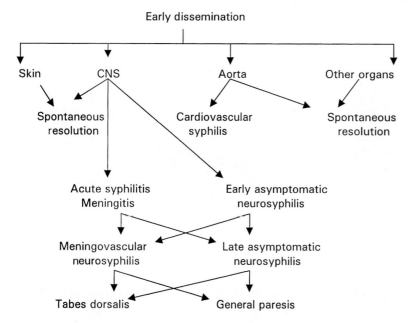

FIGURE 6.17 Pathogenesis of syphilis. (From Tramont EC. Syphilis in adults: from Christopher Columbus to Sir Alexander Fleming to AIDS. *Clin Infect Dis* 1995;21:1361–1371, with permission.)

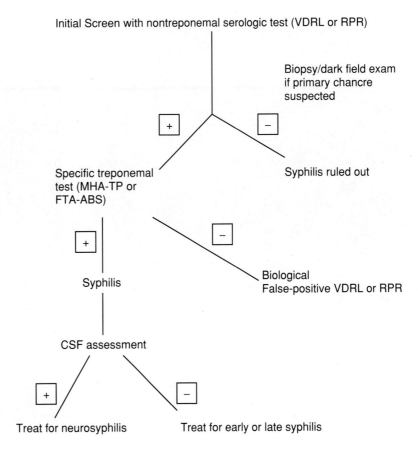

FIGURE 6.18 Diagnosis of syphilis.

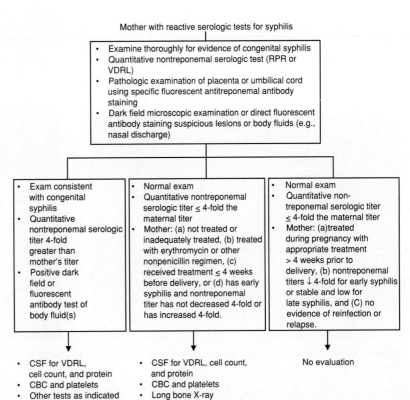

FIGURE 6.19 Diagnosis of congenital syphilis.

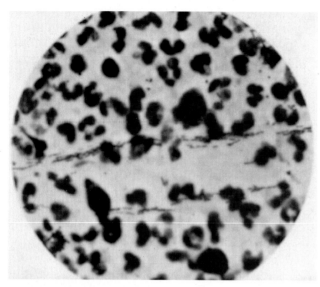

FIGURE 6.20 School of fish appearance on Gram stain of *Haemophilus ducreyi.*

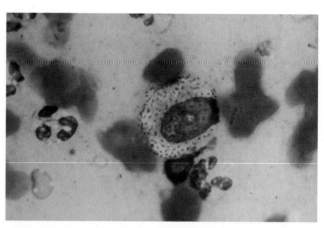

FIGURE 6.22 *Calymmatobacterium granulomatis* (Donovan body), the etiologic agent granuloma inguinale.

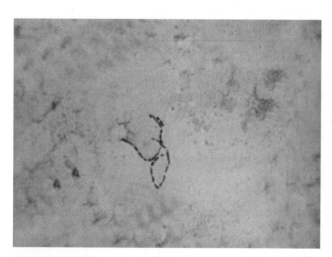

FIGURE 6.21 "School of fish" appearance of *Haemophilus ducreyi* on Gram stain.

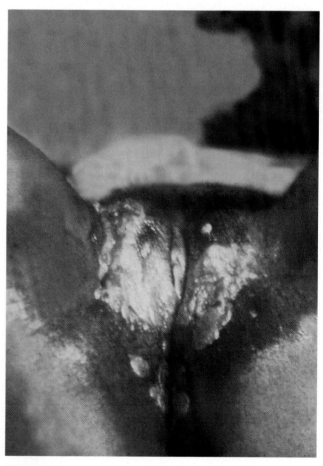

FIGURE 6.23 Granuloma inguinale.

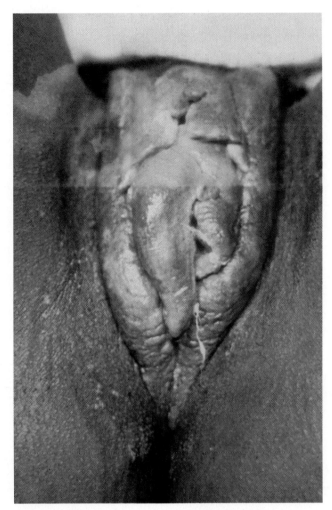

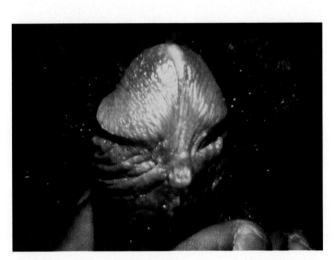

FIGURE 6.24 Primary lesion of lymphogranuloma venereum.

FIGURE 6.25 Lymphogranuloma venereum of vulva.

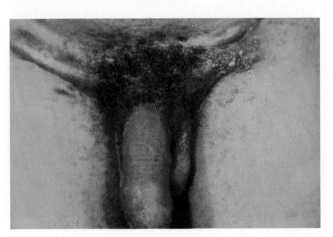

FIGURE 6.26 Grooved nodes (saddle nodes) characteristic of lymphogranuloma venereum.

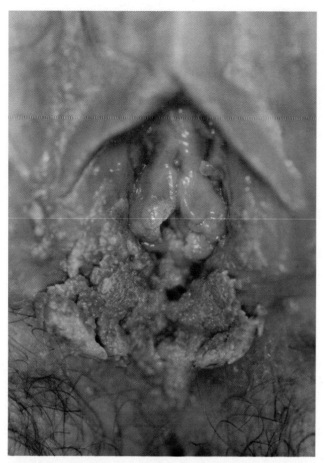

FIGURE 6.27 Vaginal and perineal genital warts of human papilloma virus (HPV).

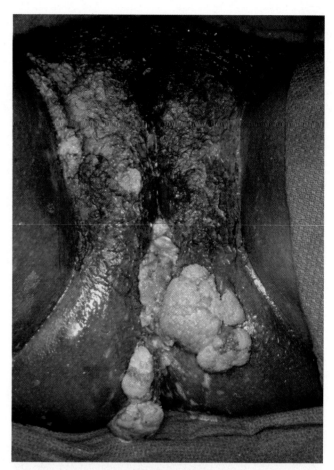

FIGURE 6.29 Genital warts (condyloma acuminatum).

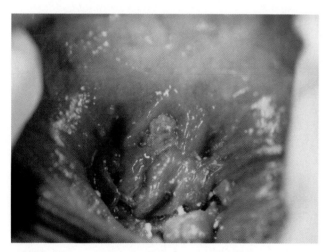

FIGURE 6.28 Urethral genital warts of HPV.

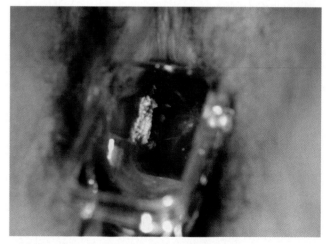

FIGURE 6.30 Genital warts of vaginal wall.

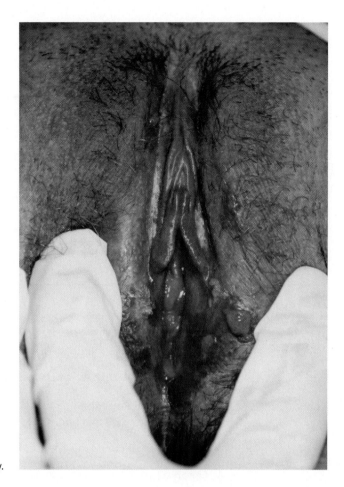

FIGURE 6.31 Genital warts post–laser therapy.

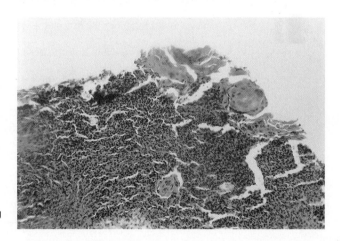

FIGURE 6.32 Molluscum contagiosum. Microscopic view showing typical molluscum bodies as well as inflammation.

BOX 6.1

Recommended Regimens for Pediculosis Pubis (Pubic Lice)

- **Permethrin 1% cream rinse** applied to affected areas and washed off after 10 minutes
  or
- **Lindane 1% shampoo** applied for 4 minutes to affected area and then thoroughly washed off (NOT recommended for pregnant or lactating women or children aged <2 years)
  or
- **Pyrethrins with piperonyl butoxide** applied to affected area and washed off after 10 minutes

Note: From Centers for Disease Control and Prevention. Sexually transmitted diseases treatment guidelines. *MMWR* 2002;51 (RR-6):1–78, with permission.

BOX 6.2

Recommended Regimens for Scabies

Recommended Regimen
- **Permethrin cream (5%)** applied to all areas of body from neck down and washed off after 8–14 hours

Alternative Regimen
- **Lindane (1%)** l oz. of lotion or 30 g cream applied in a thin layer to all areas of body from neck down and thoroughly washed off after 8 hours (should not be used in pregnant or lactating women, children <2 years, or patients with extensive dermatitis)
  or
- **Ivermectin** 200 mcg/kg, repeated in 2 weeks

Note: From Centers for Disease Control and Prevention. Sexually transmitted diseases treatment guidelines. *MMWR* 2002; 51 (RR-6):1–78, with permission.

BOX 6.3

Recommended Regimens for Uncomplicated Gonococcal Infections of the Cervix, Urethra, and Rectum in Adults

Recommended Regimen
- Cefixime 400 mg PO in a single dose
  or
- Ceftriaxone 125 mg IM in a single dose
  or
- Ciprofloxacin 500 mg PO in a single dose
  or
- Ofloxacin 400 mg PO in a single dose
  or
- Levofloxacin 250 mg PO in a single dose
  plus
- Azithromycin 1 g PO in a single dose
  or
- Doxycycline 100 mg PO b.i.d. for 7 days

Alternative Regimen
- Spectinomycin 2 g IM in a single dose
- Single-dose cephalosporins such as ceftizoxime 500 mg IM, cefotaxime 500 mg IM, cefotetan 1 g IM, and cefoxitin 2 g IM with probenecid 1 g PO.
- Single dose other quinolones such as gatifloxacin 400 mg PO, lomefloxacin 400 mg PO, or norfloxacin 800 mg PO.

Note: From Centers for Disease Control and Prevention. Sexually transmitted diseases treatment guidelines. *MMWR* 2002;51(RR-6):1–78, with permission.

BOX 6.4
Recommended Regimens for Disseminated Gonococcal Infection

Recommended Initial Regimen
- Ceftriaxone 1 g IM or IV every 24 hours

Alternative Initial Regimen
- Cefotaxime 1 g IV every 8 hours
  or
- Ceftizoxime 1 g IV every 8 hours
  or

For persons allergic to β-lactam drugs:
- Ciprofloxacin 500 mg IV every 12 hours
  or
- Ofloxacin 400 mg IV every 12 hours or Levofloxacin 250 mg IV daily
  or
- Spectinomycin 2 g IM every 12 hours

All regimens should be continued for 24–48 hours after improvement begins, at which time, therapy may be switched to one of the following regimens to complete a full week of therapy:
- Cefixime 400 mg PO b.i.d.
  or
- Ciprofloxacin 500 mg PO b.i.d.[a]
  or
- Ofloxacin 400 mg PO b.i.d.[a] or Levofloxacin 500 mg PO daily

---

[a]Ciprofloxacin and ofloxacin are contraindicated in pregnant or lactating women.
Note: From Centers for Disease Control and Prevention. Sexually transmitted diseases treatment guidelines. *MMWR* 2002;51(RR-6):1–78, with permission.

BOX 6.5
Recommended Regimens for Syphilis in Adults

Early Syphilis (primary, secondary and early latent)
Recommended Regimen
- Benzathine penicillin G, 2.4 million units IM in a single dose

Penicillin Allergy (nonpregnant)[a]
- Doxycycline 100 mg PO b.i.d. for 2 weeks
  or
- Tetracycline 500 mg PO q.i.d. for 2 weeks

Late Syphilis (late latent and tertiary)
Recommended Regimen
- Benzathine penicillin G, 7.2 million units IM total, administered as 3 doses of 2.4 million units IM at 1-week intervals

Penicillin Allergy (nonpregnant)
- Doxycycline 100 mg PO b.i.d. for 4 weeks
  or
- Tetracycline 500 mg PO q.i.d. for 4 weeks

---

[a]Limited clinical studies suggest that ceftriaxone 1 g daily IM or IV for 8–10 days or azithromycin as single oral dose of 2 g are effective for treatment of early syphilis.
Note: From Centers for Disease Control and Prevention. Sexually transmitted diseases treatment guidelines. *MMWR* 2002;51(RR-6):1–78, with permission.

BOX 6.6
Recommended Regimens for Syphilis in Pregnant Women

Recommended Regimen
- Penicillin regimen appropriate for the stage of syphilis

Penicillin Allergy[a]
- Desensitize and treat with penicillin

[a]No alternatives to penicillin have been proved effective for treatment of syphilis in pregnancy.
Note: From Centers for Disease Control and Prevention. Sexually transmitted diseases treatment guidelines. *MMWR* 2002;51 (RR-6):1–78, with permission.

BOX 6.8
Recommended Regimens for Donovanosis (Granuloma Inguinale)

Recommended Regimen
- Trimethoprim-sulfamethoxazole one double-strength tablet PO b.i.d. for a minimum of 3 weeks
  or
- Doxycycline 100 mg PO b.i.d. for a minimum of 3 weeks

Alternative Regimen
- Ciprofloxacin 750 mg PO b.i.d. for a minimum of 3 weeks
  or
- Erythromycin base 500 mg PO q.i.d. for a minimum of 3 weeks
  or
- Azithromycin 1 g PO once per week for at least 3 weeks

Note: From Centers for Disease Control and Prevention. Sexually transmitted diseases treatment guidelines. *MMWR* 2002;51 (RR-6):1–78, with permission.

BOX 6.7
Recommended Regimens for Neurosyphilis

Recommended Regimen
- Aqueous crystalline penicillin, 18–24 million units daily, administered as 3–4 million units IV every 4 hours for 10–14 days

Alternative regimen
- Procaine penicillin, 2.4 million units IM daily, plus probenecid, 500 mg PO q.i.d., both for 10 days

Penicillin Allergy
- Ceftriaxone 2 g daily IM or IV for 10–14 days
  or
- Desensitize and treat with penicillin

Note: From Centers for Disease Control and Prevention. Sexually transmitted diseases treatment guidelines. *MMWR* 2002;51 (RR-6):1–78, with permission.

BOX 6.9
Recommended Regimens for Lymphogranuloma Venereum

Recommended Regimen
- Doxycycline 100 mg PO b.i.d. for 21 days
  or

Alternative Regimen
- Erythromycin 500 mg PO q.i.d. for 21 days

Note: From Centers for Disease Control and Prevention. Sexually transmitted diseases treatment guidelines. *MMWR* 2002;51 (RR-6):I–78, with permission.

BOX 6.10
Recommended Regimens for External Genital Warts

Recommended Regimen

Patient-applied:

- **Podofilox 0.5% solution or gel,**[a] applied with a cotton swab (solution), or with a finger (gel), to visible genital warts b.i.d. for 3 days, followed by 4 days of no therapy. Cycle may be repeated as necessary for a total of four cycles.

   or

- **Imiquimod 5% cream,**[a] applied with finger at bedtime t.i.w. for up to 16 weeks

Provider-administered:

- **Cryotherapy** with liquid nitrogen or cryoprobe; repeat every I to 2 weeks

   or

- **Podophyllin resin 10–25%**[a] in compound tincture or benzoin; repeat weekly if necessary

   or

- **Trichloracetic acid or bichloracetic acid 80–90%;** repeat weekly if necessary

   or

- **Surgical removal** by tangential scissor excision, tangential shave excision, curettage, or electrosurgery

Alternative Regimen

- Intralesional interferon

   or

- Laser surgery

---

[a]Should not be used during pregnancy.
Note: From Centers for Disease Control and Prevention. Sexually transmitted diseases treatment guidelines. *MMWR* 2002;51(RR-6):1–78, with permission.

BOX 6.11
Recommended Regimens for Vaginal, Urethral, and Anal Genital Warts

Recommended Regimen Vaginal Warts

- **Cryotherapy** with liquid nitrogen

   or

- **TCA or BCA 80%–90%**

Recommended Regimen Urethral Meatus Warts

- **Cryotherapy** with liquid nitrogen

   or

- **Podophyllin**[a] **10–25%** in tincture benzoin

Recommended Regimen Anal Warts

- **Cryotherapy** with liquid nitrogen

   or

- **TCA or BCA 80%–90%**

   or

- **Surgical removal**

---

[a]Should not be used during pregnancy.
Note: From Centers for Disease Control and Prevention. Sexually transmitted diseases treatment guidelines. *MMWR* 2002;51(RR-6):1–78, with permission.

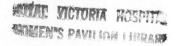

BOX 6.12

Recommended Regimens for Chancroid

Recommended Regimen

- Azithromycin 1 g PO in a single dose
    or
- Ceftriaxone 250 mg IM in a single dose
    or
- Ciprofloxacin[a] 500 mg PO b.i.d. for 3 days
    or
- Erythromycin base 500 mg PO q.i.d. for 7 days

---

[a]Contraindicated for pregnant and lactating women.
Note: From Centers for Disease Control and Prevention. Sexually transmitted diseases treatment guidelines. *MMWR* 2002;51(RR-6):1–78, with permission.

7

MIXED ANAEROBIC-AEROBIC PELVIC INFECTION AND PELVIC ABSCESS

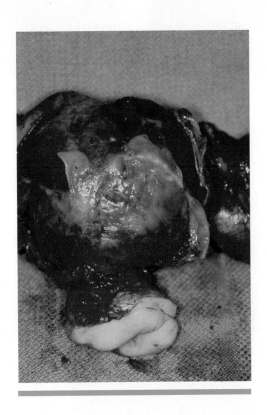

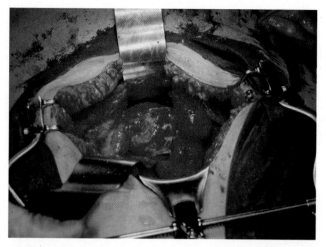

FIGURE 7.1 Tuboovarian abscess at exploratory laparotomy.

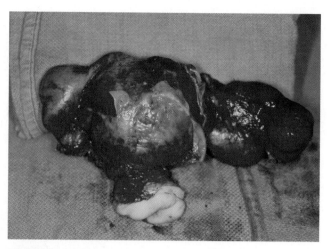

FIGURE 7.2 Tuboovarian abscess.

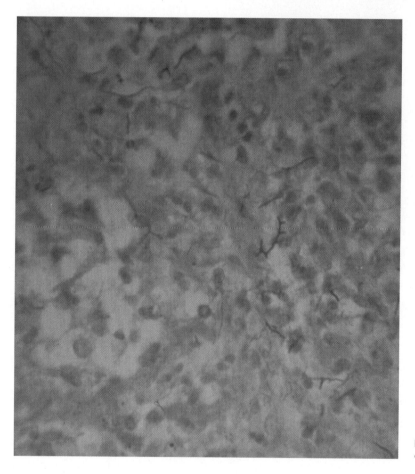

FIGURE 7.3 *Actinomyces israelii* in wall of tuboovarian abscess.

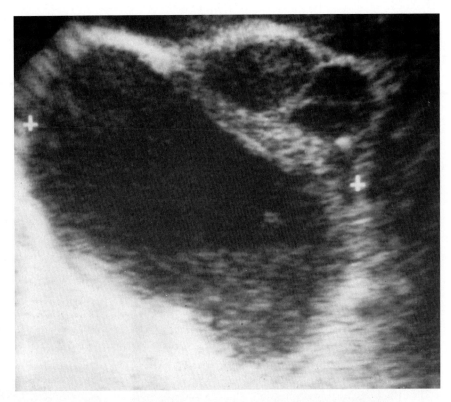

FIGURE 7.4 Ultrasound image of tuboovarian abscess.

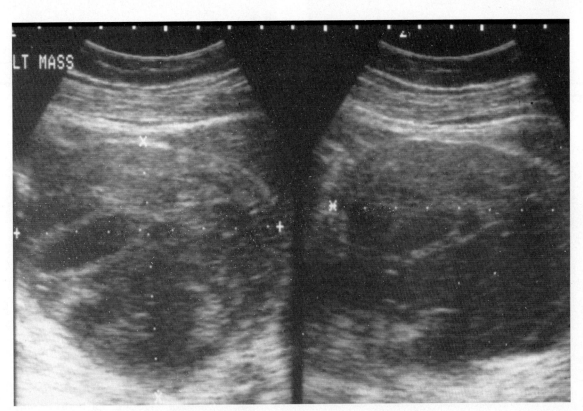

FIGURE 7.5 Ultrasound of tuboovarian abscess.

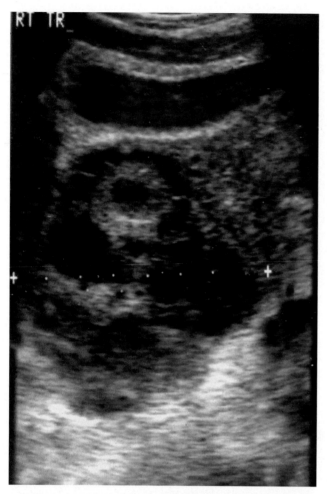

FIGURE 7.6 Ultrasound demonstrating tuboovarian abscess.

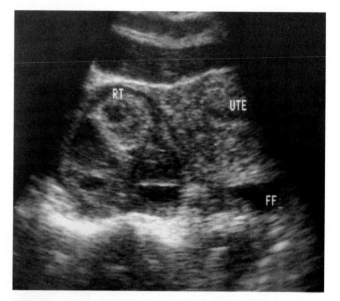

FIGURE 7.7 Ultrasound image of tuboovarian abscess.

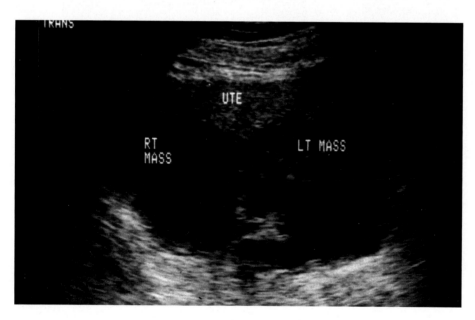

FIGURE 7.8 Ultrasound demonstrating bilateral tuboovarian abscesses.

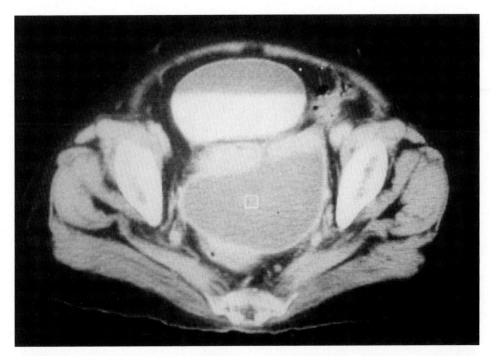

FIGURE 7.9 CT scan of tuboovarian abscess.

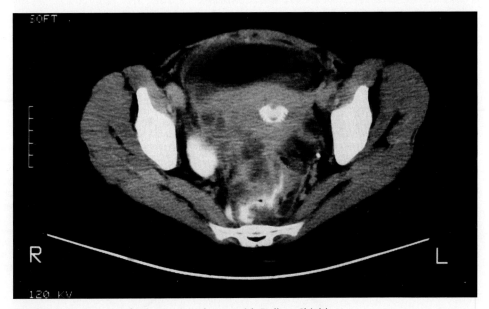

FIGURE 7.10 CT scan of tuboovarian abscess with Dalkon Shield.

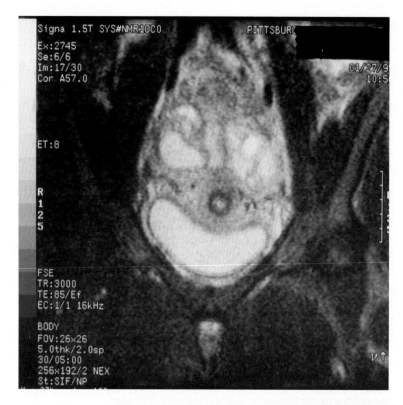

FIGURE 7.11 MRI tuboovarian abscess.

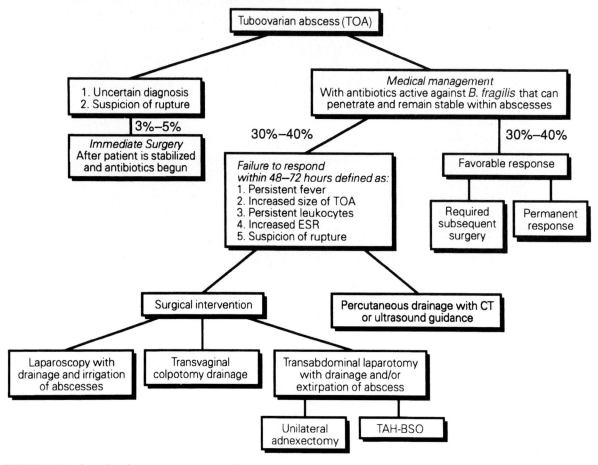

FIGURE 7.12 Algorithm for the management of tuboovarian abscesses.

8

HEPATITIS INFECTION

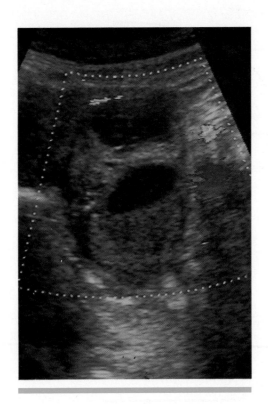

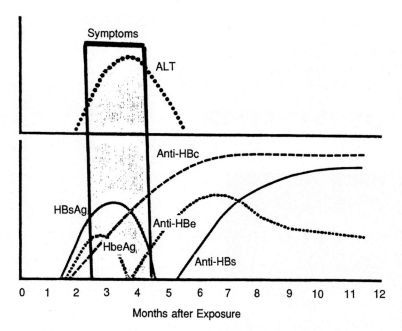

FIGURE 8.1 Serologic pattern in patients with acute hepatitis B that resolves.

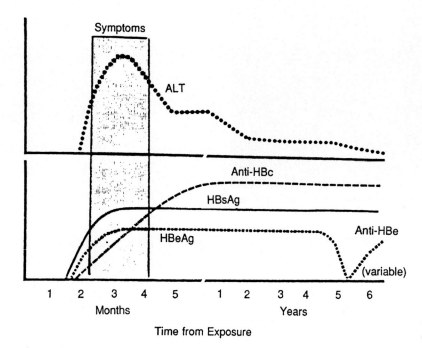

FIGURE 8.2 Serologic pattern in patients with chronic hepatitis B.

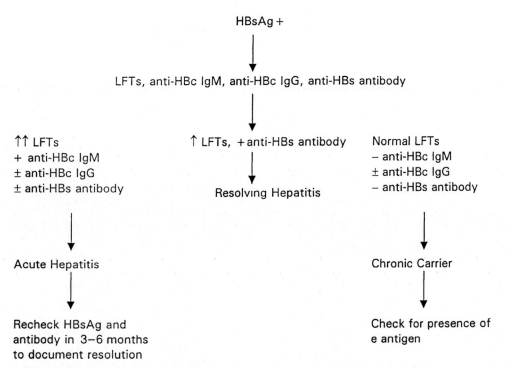

FIGURE 8.3 Algorithm for evaluation of HBsAg-positive patients. HBsAg, hepatitis B surface antigen; anti-HBs, antibody to hepatitis B surface antigen; anti-HBc, antibody to hepatitis B core antigen; LFTs, liver function tests. (From Dinsmoor MJ. Hepatitis in the obstetric patient. *Infect Dis Clin North Am* 1997;11:77–91, with permission).

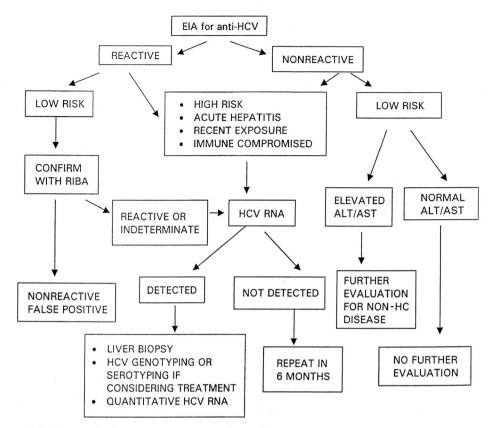

FIGURE 8.4 Algorithm for diagnosis of hepatitis C infection. EIA, enzyme immunoassay; HCV, hepatitis C virus; RIBA, recombinant immunoblot assay; ALT, alanine aminotransferase; AST, aspartate aminotransferase. (From Thomas DL, Lemon SM. Hepatitis. In: Mandel GL, Bennett JE, Dolm R, eds. *Principles and practice of infectious diseases.* New York: Churchill Livingstone, 2000:1736–1760; and Schiff ER, Medina MD, Kahn RS. New perspectives in the diagnosis of hepatitis C. *Semin Liver Dis* 1999;19:3–15, with permission.)

BOX 8.1

Groups at Increased Risk of Hepatitis B Virus Infection and for Whom Hepatitis B Vaccine is Recommended

- Medical, dental, laboratory workers, and others with exposure to human blood
- Men who have sex with men
- Heterosexuals with multiple sex partners or with sexually transmitted diseases
- High HBV-endemic populations (e.g., Alaskan natives)
- Household contacts of HBsAg-positive persons
- Parenteral drug users
- Hemophilia patients
- Hemodialysis patients
- Patients for whom multiple blood/blood product infusions are anticipated
- Prison inmates and staff
- Patients and staff of institutions for mentally disabled
- Travelers to high HBV-endemic areas with anticipated exposure to blood, sexual contacts with locals, or prolonged residence in household with locals
- Newborn infants of serum HBsAg-positive mothers[a]

HBV, hepatitis B virus; HBsAg, hepatitis B surface antigen
[a] All newborns should receive hepatitis B vaccine.
Note: From Centers for Disease Control and Prevention. Protection against viral hepatitis. Recommendations of the Advisory Committee on Immunization Practices (ACIP). *MMWR Morb Mortal Wkly Rep* 1990;39 (No. RR-2): 1–26; Advisory Committee on Immunization Practices (ACIP). Hepatitis B virus: a comparative strategy for eliminating transmission in the United States through universal childhood vaccination. *MMWR Morb Mortal Wkly Rep* 1991;40 (No. RR-13): 1–25, with permission.

BOX 8.2

Persons for Whom Screening for Hepatitis C Virus (HCV) Infection Should be Undertaken

Persons tested routinely for HCV infection
- Ever injected illegal drugs
- Selected medical conditions
  received clotting factor concentrates produced before 1987
  ever on chronic hemodialysis
  persistently elevated alanine aminotransferase levels
- Prior recipients of transfusions or organ transplants
  Notified received blood from donor who later tested positive for HCV
  Received transfusion blood or blood components before July 1992
  Received organ transplant before July 1992
- Health care, emergency medical, and public safety workers after needle sticks, sharps, or mucosal exposures to HCV-positive blood
- Children born to HCV-positive women

Persons for whom routine testing for HCV Infection is uncertain
- Recipients of transplanted tissue (e.g., corneal, skin, ova, sperm)
- Intranasal cocaine and other noninjecting illegal drug users
- History of tattooing or body piercing
- History of multiple sex partners
- History of sexually transmitted diseases
- Long-term steady sex partner of HCV-positive person(s)

Note: From Centers for Disease Control and Prevention.
Recommendations for prevention and control of hepatitis C virus (HCV) infection and HCV-related chronic disease. *MMWR Morb Mortal Wkly Rep* 1998;47 (No. RR-19): 1–39, with permission.

GYNECOLOGIC AND OBSTETRIC INFECTIONS

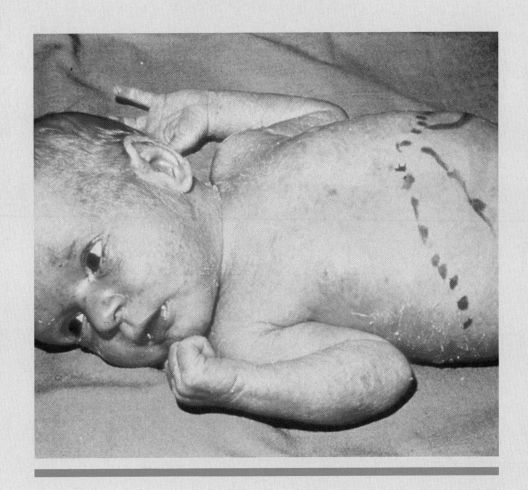

9

TOXIC SHOCK SYNDROME

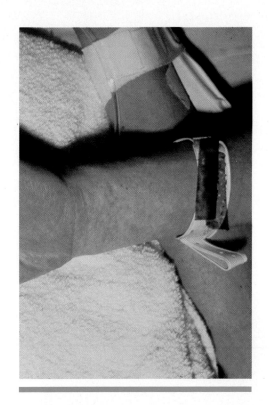

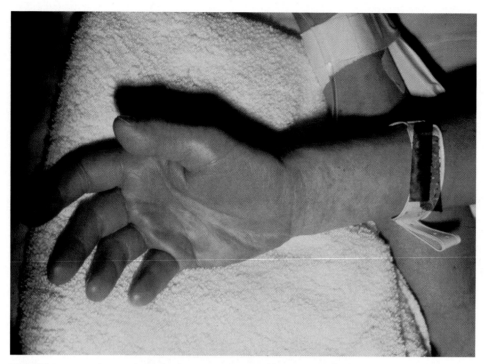

FIGURE 9.1 Macular erythematous rash of staphylococcal toxic shock syndrome.

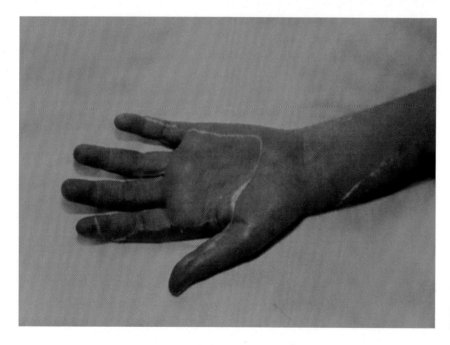

FIGURE 9.2 Desquamation of rash post-staphylococcal toxic shock syndrome.

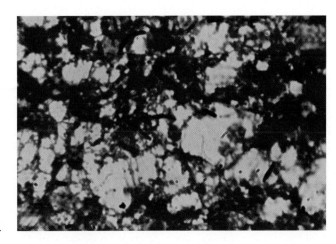

FIGURE 9.3 Gram stain of *Clostridium sordellii*.

BOX 9.1
Case Definition of Toxic Shock Syndrome

1. Fever (temperature ≥38.9°C, 102°F)
2. Rash characterized by diffuse macular erythro-derma
3. Desquamation occurring 1–2 weeks after onset of illness (in survivors)
4. Hypotension (systolic blood pressure ≤90 mm Hg in adults) or orthostatic syncope
5. Involvement of three or more of the following organ systems:
   a. Gastrointestinal (vomiting or diarrhea at onset of illness)
   b. Muscular (myalgia or creatine phosphokinase level twice normal)
   c. Mucous membrane (vaginal, oropharyngeal, or conjunctival hyperemia)
   d. Renal (blood urea nitrogen or creatinine level ≥ twice normal or ≥5 white blood cells per high-power field in absence of urinary tract infection)
   e. Hepatic (total bilirubin, serum glutamic-oxaloacetic transaminase [SGOT] or serum glutamic-pyruvic transaminase [SGPT] twice normal level)
   f. Hematologic (platelets ≤100,000/mm³)
   g. Central nervous system (disorientation or alterations in consciousness without focal neurologic signs when fever and hypotension absent)
   h. Cardiopulmonary (adult respiratory distress syndrome, pulmonary edema, new onset of second- or third-degree heart block, myocarditis)
6. Negative throat and cerebrospinal fluid cultures (apositive blood culture for *Staphylococcus aureus* does not exclude a case)
7. Negative serologic tests for Rocky Mountain spotted fever, leptospirosis, rubeola

Note: From Toxic shock syndrome—United States, 1970–1982. *MMWR* 1982; 31:201.

BOX 9.2
Proposed Case Definition for Streptococcal Toxic Shock Syndrome[a]

I. Isolation of group A streptococci (*Streptococcus pyogenes*)
   A. From a normally sterile site (e.g., blood; cerebrospinal, pleural, or peritoneal fluid; tissue biopsy; surgical wound)
   B. From a nonsterile site (e.g., throat, sputum, vagina, superficial skin lesion)
II. Clinical signs of severity
   A. Hypotension: systolic BP ≤90 mm Hg in adults or less than fifth percentile for age in children *and*
   B. ≥2 of the following signs:
      1. Renal impairment: creatinine ≥177 uM (≥2 mg/dL)
      2. Coagulopathy: ≤100 × 10⁹/L (≤100,000/mm³) or disseminated intravascular coagulation (prolonged clotting time, low fibrinogen levels, and presence of fibrin degradation products)
      3. Liver involvement: serum glutamic-oxaloacetic transaminase (SGOT), serum glutamic-pyruvic transaminase (SGPT), or total bilirubin twice or greater than upper limits of normal
      4. Adult respiratory distress syndrome
      5. Generalized erythematous macular rash that may desquamate
      6. Soft tissue necrosis (necrotizing fasciitis, myositis, or gangrene)

[a] An illness fulfilling criteria IA and II (A and B) is defined as a *definite* case. An illness fulfilling criteria IB and II (A and B) is defined as a *probable* case if no other etiology for the illness is identified.

10

INFECTIOUS VULVOVAGINITIS

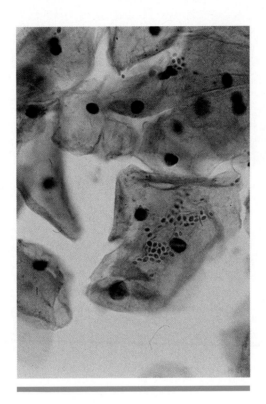

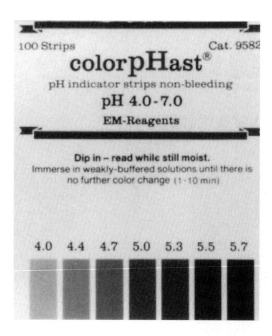

FIGURE 10.1 pH paper used in the differential diagnosis of vulvovaginitis. The pH range is from 4.0 to 7.0.

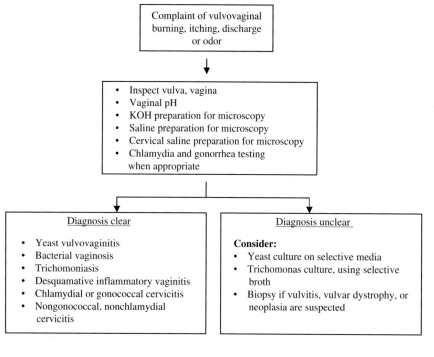

FIGURE 10.2 Algorithm for patients complaining of vulvovaginal burning, itching, discharge, or odor. (See Table 10-1 on page 77.)

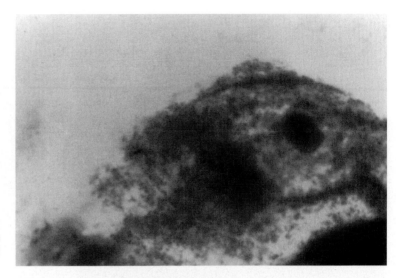

FIGURE 10.3 Vaginal Gram stain showing a true clue cell and abnormal bacteria characteristic of bacterial vaginosis.

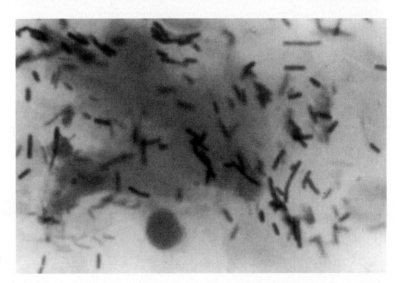

FIGURE 10.4 Gram stain showing normal vaginal flora with a predominance of *Lactobacillus* morphotypes.

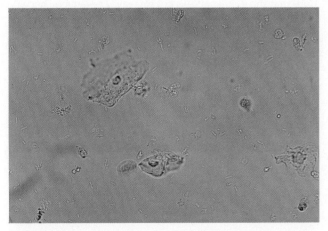

FIGURE 10.5 Normal wet mount showing few epithelial cells, rare white blood cells, and rods characteristic of lactobacilli.

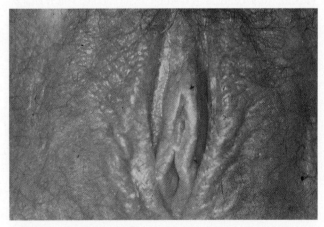

FIGURE 10.6 Candida vulvitis. Note the edema and erythema.

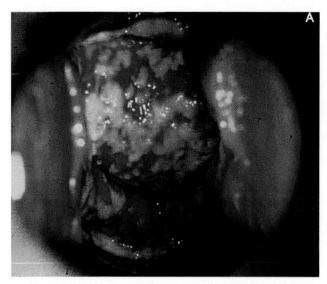

FIGURE 10.7 Candida vaginitis. Note the adherent white "cottage cheese" type discharge.

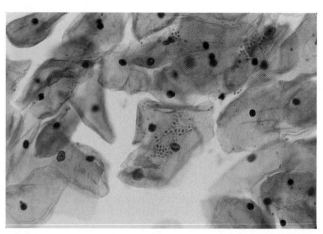

FIGURE 10.9 *Candida glabrata* as seen on a Papanicolaou smear. Buds are seen without pseudohyphae. This finding suggests *non–Candida albicans* species.

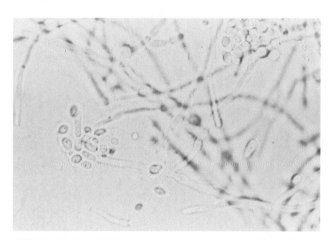

FIGURE 10.8 Candida as seen on a wet mount. This is characteristic of *Candida albicans*.

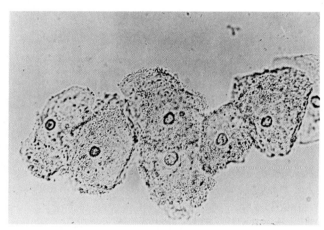

FIGURE 10.10 Wet mount showing characteristic clue cells. Note that the epithelial cells are so heavily covered by bacteria as to obscure the margins.

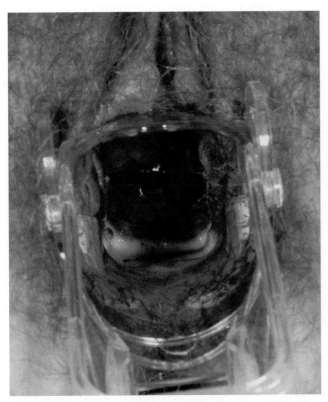

FIGURE 10.11 Homogeneous vaginal discharge of bacterial vaginosis.

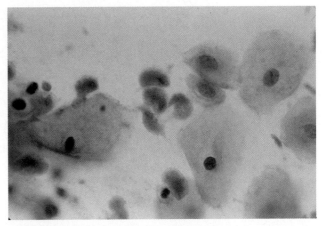

FIGURE 10.12 Papanicolaou smear showing *Trichomonas vaginalis*. Note the cell with the characteristic shape of a trichomonad in the center of the photograph.

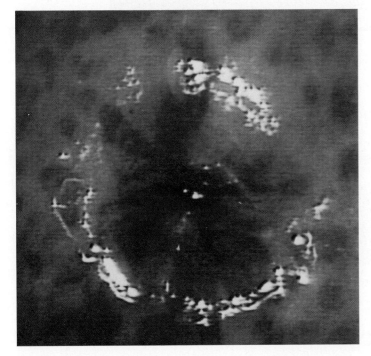

FIGURE 10.13 Strawberry cervix associated with trichomoniasis.

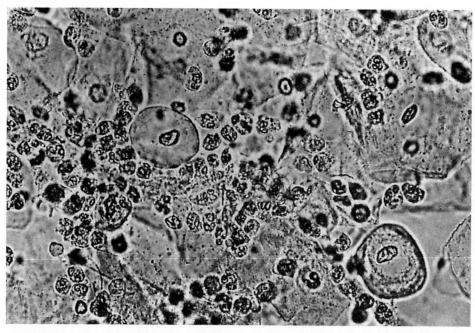

FIGURE 10.14 Wet-mount findings in desquamative inflammatory vaginitis. Note the abundant polymorphonuclear leukocytes and parabasal cells. (From Paavonen J. *J Infect Dis Obstet* 1996;4:257, with permission.)

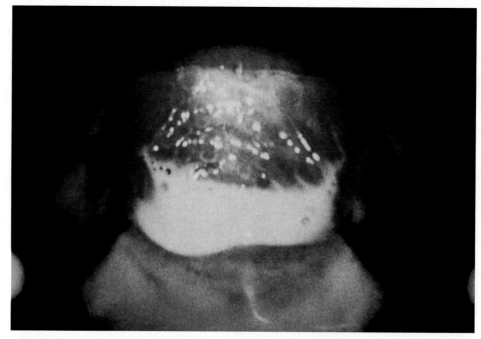

FIGURE 10.15 Desquamative inflammatory vaginitis. (From Paavonen, J. *J Infect Dis Obstet* 1996;4:257, with permission.)

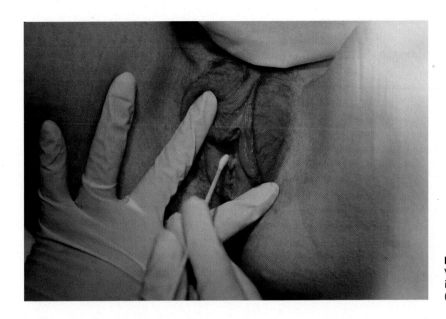

FIGURE 10.16 Vulvar Vestibulitis Syndrome, Vulvodynia. Characteristic physical findings include exquisite tenderness to light pressure (such as with a Qtip) in vaginal vestibule.

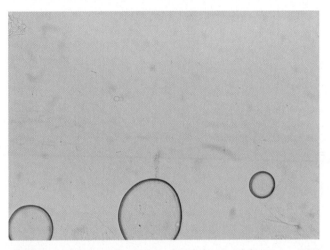

FIGURE 10.17 Round spheres of *Torulopsis glabrata* on KOH smear.

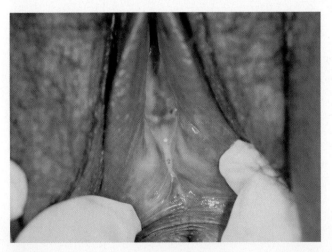

FIGURE 10.18 Homogeneous discharge of bacterial vaginosis.

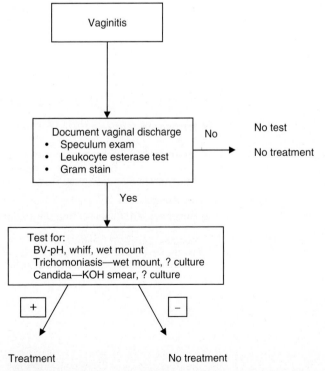

Vaginitis

Document vaginal discharge
- Speculum exam
- Leukocyte esterase test
- Gram stain

No → No test / No treatment

Yes ↓

Test for:
BV-pH, whiff, wet mount
Trichomoniasis—wet mount, ? culture
Candida—KOH smear, ? culture

+ → Treatment

− → No treatment

FIGURE 10.19 Follow up if symptoms recur or persist. (Vulvovaginitis)

BOX 10.1

Classification of Vulvovaginal Candidiasis (VVC)

Uncomplicated VVC
- Sporadic or infrequent vulvovaginal candidiasis
  or
- Mild to moderate vulvovaginal candidiasis
  or
- Likely to be *C. albicans*
  or
- Nonimmunocompromised women

Complicated VVC
- Recurrent vulvovaginal candidiasis
  or
- Severe vulvovaginal candidiasis
  or
- Nonalbicans candidiasis
  or
- Women with uncontrolled diabetes, debilitation, or immunosuppression, or those who are pregnant

---

BOX 10.2

Recommended Regimens

Intravaginal Agents
- **Butoconazole** 2% cream 5 g intravaginally q.d. for 3 days[a]
  or
- **Butoconazole** 2% cream 5 g (Butaconazole 1-sustained release), single intravaginal application
  or
- **Clotrimazole** 1% cream 5 g intravaginally q.d. for 7–14 days[a]
  or
- **Clotrimazole** 100 mg vaginal tablet q.d. for 7 days
  or
- **Clotrimazole** 100 mg vaginal tablet, two tablets q.d. for 3 days
  or
- **Clotrimazole** 500 mg vaginal tablet, single intravaginal application
  or
- **Miconazole** 2% cream 5 g intravaginally q.d. for 7 days[a]
  or
- **Miconazole** 100 mg vaginal suppository q.d. for 7 days[a]
  or
- **Miconazole** 200 mg vaginal suppository q.d. for 3 days[a]
  or
- **Nystatin** 100,000-unit vaginal tablet q.d. 14 days
  or
- **Tioconazole** 6.5% ointment 5 g, single intravaginal application[a]
  or
- **Terconazole** 0.4% cream 5 g intravaginally q.d. for 7 days
  or
- **Terconazole** 0.8% cream 5 g intravaginally q.d. for 3 days
  or
- **Terconazole** 80 mg vaginal suppository q.d. for 3 days

Oral Agent
- **Fluconazole** 150 mg PO in a single dose.

---

[a] Over-the-counter (OTC) preparations.
Note: The creams and suppositories in this regimen are based and may weaken latex condoms and diaphragms. Refer to condom product labeling for further information.

BOX 10.3

Treatment and Prevention of Recurrent Vulvovaginal Candidiasis[a]

Step 1: Eradication Regimen
- Fluconazole 150 mg PO on days 1, 4, and 8
  or
- Intravaginal azoles for 10–14 days
  or
- Ketoconazole 400 mg q.d. for 14 days

Step 2: Prevention Regimen for 3–6 months
- Fluconazole 150 mg PO weekly
  or
- Ketoconazole 100 mg PO daily
  or
- Itraconazole 100 mg PO every other day
  or
- Clotrimazole 500 mg vaginally weekly
  or
- Any topical azole, applied daily

[a]Recurrent candidiasis is usually defined as ≥4 episodes per year. Based on CDC 2002 STD treatment guidelines.
Note: From Sobel JD. Pathogenesis and treatment of recurrent vulvovaginal candidiasis. *Clin Infect Dis* 1992;14(Suppl 1)S148–S153; and Rex JH, Walsh TJ, Sobel JD, et al. Practice guidelines for the treatment of candidiasis. *Clin Infect Dis* 2000;30:662–678, with permission.

BOX 10.4

Clinical Criteria for Diagnosis of Bacterial Vaginosis

Presence of three of the following four criteria is necessary for diagnosis:
- Homogeneous, milky or creamy discharge
- Presence of true clue cells on microscopic examination
- pH of secretions >4.5
- Fishy or amine odor with or without addition of 10% KOH

Note: From CDC 2002. Guidelines for STD treatment. *MMWR* 2002; 51 (No. RR-6):42, with permission.

BOX 10.5

Recommended Regimens for Bacterial Vaginosis in Non-Pregnant Women

Recommended Regimen
- Metronidazole 500 mg PO b.i.d. for 7 days
  or
- Metronidazole 0.75% gel 5 g intravaginally q.d. for 5 days
  or
- Clindamycin 2% cream 5 g intravaginally q.n. for 7 days.

Alternative Regimen
- Metronidazole 2 g PO in a single dose
  or
- Clindamycin 300 mg PO b.i.d. for 7 days
  or
- Clindamycin ovules 100 g intravaginally q.n. for 3 days

Note: From CDC 2002 Guidelines for Treatment of STDs. *MMWR* 2002;51(No. RR-6):43, with permission.

BOX 10.6

Recommended Regimens for Bacterial Vaginosis in Pregnant Women

Recommended Regimen
- Metronidazole 250 mg PO t.i.d. for 7 days
  or
- Clindamycin 300 mg PO b.i.d. for 7 days

Note: From CDC 2002 Guidelines for Treatment of STDs. *MMWR* 2002;51(No. RR-6):44, with permission.

BOX 10.7

Other Causes of Vulvar Burning or Pruritis (Besides Candidiasis)

- Vulvar Vestibulitis Syndrome/Vulvodynia
- Lichen sclerosis
- Lichen simplex chronicus
- Contact dermatitis
- Vulvar neoplasia
- Lichen planus
- Steroid rebound dermatitis

BOX 10.9

Recommended Regimens for Trichomoniasis

Recommended Regimen
- Metronidazole 2 g PO in single dose

Alternative Regimen
- Metronidazole 500 mg PO b.i.d. for 7 days

Note: From Centers for Disease Control and Prevention. 2002 STD Treatment Guidelines. *MMWR* 2002;51(No. RR-6):44, with permission.

BOX 10.8

Recommended Regimens for Nonalbicans Candidal[a] Vulvovaginitis

- Longer duration of therapy (7–14 days) with an azole drug, other than fluconazole (first line therapy)
  or
- Boric acid, 600 mg size 0 gelatin capsules intravaginally q.d. for 14 days (highly toxic when taken orally)
  or
- Flucytosine (Ancoban) 4% cream to be applied topically (referral to a specialist is advised[b])
  or
- Nystatin 100,000-unit vaginal suppository q.d. 14–28 days (may also be useful as a maintenance regimen[b])

[a]These species are commonly *C. glabrata* or *C. tropicalis.*
[b]From CDC Sexually Transmitted Disease Treatment Guidelines. *MMWR* 2002;51(No. RR-6):47, with permission.

BOX 10.10

Characteristics of Desquamative Inflammatory Vaginitis

Diagnosis
- Heavy, often frothy discharge
- pH >4.5
- Purulent vaginitis with vaginal erythema
- Wet mounts: abundant coccoid bacteria (rare to no lactobacilli); large numbers of polymorphonuclear leukocytes and parabasal cells, but no clue cells

Differential diagnosis
- Atrophic vaginitis
- Trichomoniasis
- Erosive lichen planus
- Cervicitis
- Foreign body
- Cervical or vaginal cancer (with secondary necrosis and exudate)
- Bacterial vaginosis

Treatment
- Clindamycin vaginal cream 2%
- In estrogen-deficient women, replacement therapy may help, especially when there is relapse.

TABLE 10.1 CHARACTERISTICS OF NORMAL SECRETIONS AND VAGINITIS

Feature	Normal	Bacterial Vaginosis	Trichomoniasis	Yeast
Appearance	White; floccular high viscosity	Gray, white; milky/creamy	Gray, Yellow, greenish, or white; homogeneous, often frothy	White; often curdy
pH	<4.5	>4.5	>4.5	<4.5
Amine odor	Absent	Present	Absent	Absent
Clue cells	Absent	Present	Absent	Absent
Trichomonads	Absent	Absent	Present	Absent
Mycelia	Absent	Absent	Absent	Present

11

POSTABORTION INFECTION, BACTEREMIA, AND SEPTIC SHOCK

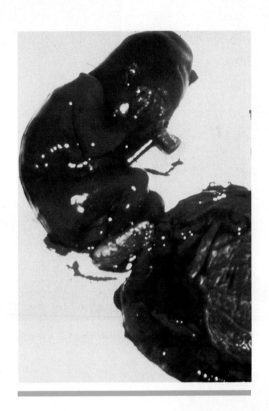

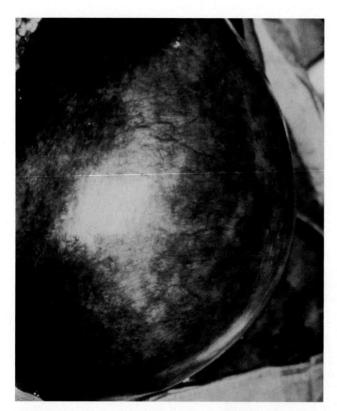

FIGURE 11.1 Clostridial "gas gangrene" of uterus.

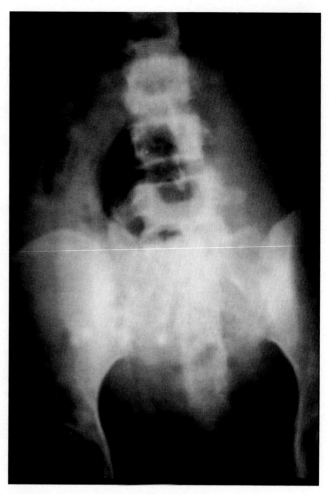

FIGURE 11.2 Clostridial "gas gangrene" of uterus (x-ray).

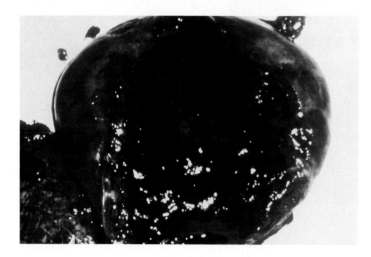

FIGURE 11.3 Clostridial myonecrosis of uterus.

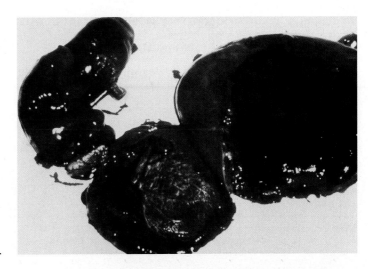

FIGURE 11.4 Septic abortion with clostridial myonecrosis.

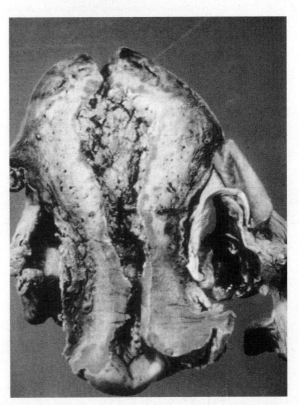

FIGURE 11.5 Uterus removed at autopsy from lethal septic abortion. Note retained products of conception and site of uterine perforation at fundus.

TABLE 11.1   DRUGS COMMONLY USED FOR CIRCULATORY SUPPORT

Drug	Pharmacologic Role	Clinical Effect	Usual Dose Range
Epinephrine	α- and β-Adrenergic agonist	Chronotropism, inotropism, vasoconstriction	5–20 μg/min
Norepinephrine	α- and β-Adrenergic agonist[a]	Chronotropism, inotropism, vasoconstriction	5–20 μg/min
Dopamine	Dopamine and β-adrenergic agonist, progressive α-adrenergic effect with increasing doses	Chronotropism, inotropism, vasoconstriction	2–20 μg/kg body weight/min
Dobutamine	β-Adrenergic agonist	Chronotropism, inotropism, vasodilation	5–15 μg/kg/min
Phenylephrine	α-Adrenergic agonist	Vasoconstriction	2–20 μg/min

[a] The α-adrenergic effect is greater than the β-adrenergic effect.
Note: From Wheeler AP, Bernard GR. Treating patients with severe sepsis. *N Engl J Med* 1999;340:207–214, with permission.

BOX 11.1

Definitions of Systemic Inflammatory Response Syndrome[a] and Sepsis

Definition of systemic inflammatory response syndrome (SIRS)

Two or more of the following clinical signs of systemic response to endothelial inflammation:

- Temperature >38°C or <36°C
- Elevated heart rate >90 beats/min
- Tachypnea, manifested by a respiratory rate >20 breaths/min or hyperventilation, as indicated by P_aco_2 <32 mm Hg
- Altered white blood cell count >12.0 cells $\times 10^9$/L, <4.0 cells $\times 10^9$/L, or presence of >10% immature neutrophils ("bands")
- In the setting (or strong suspicion) of a known cause of endothelial inflammation, such as:

    Infection (caused by Gram-negative or Gram-positive bacteria, viruses, fungi, parasites, yeasts, or other organisms)
    Pancreatitis
    Ischemia
    Multiple trauma and tissue injury
    Hemorrhagic shock
    Immune-mediated organ injury
    Administration of an exogenous mediate (e.g., tumor necrosis factor, interleukin-1, interleukin-2)

- In the absence of any other known cause of such clinical abnormalities

Definition of Sepsis

In association with infection, manifestations of sepsis are the same as those defined for SIRS and include, but are not limited to, more than one of the following:

- Temperature >38°C or <36°C
- Elevated heart rate >90 beats/min
- Tachypnea, manifested by a respiratory rate >20 breaths/min or hyperventilation, as indicated by a P_aco_2 <32 mm Hg
- Altered white blood cell count >12.0 cells $\times 10^9$/L, <4.0 cells $\times 10^9$/L, or the presence of >10% immature neutrophils ("bands")

These physiologic changes should represent an acute alteration from baseline in the absence of other known causes for such abnormalities.

---

[a] Severe SIRS and severe sepsis are defined as SIRS or sepsis associated with organ dysfunction, hypoperfusion abnormality, or inflammation-induced hypotension. Hypoperfusion abnormalities include lactic acidosis, oliguria, or acute alteration of mental status. The severity of the physiologic abnormality should be analyzed by a severity-of-illness scoring system.
Note: From Bone RC. Toward an epidemiology and natural history of SIRS (systemic inflammatory response syndrome). *JAMA* 1992;268:3452–3455, with permission.

12

PELVIC INFLAMMATORY DISEASE

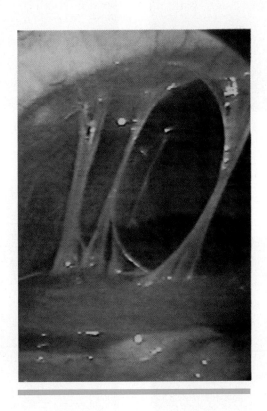

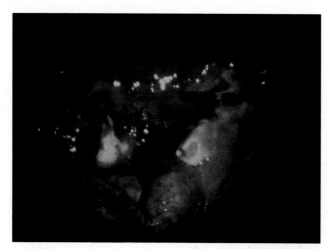

FIGURE 12.1 Laparoscopic view of acute pelvic inflammatory disease (PID).

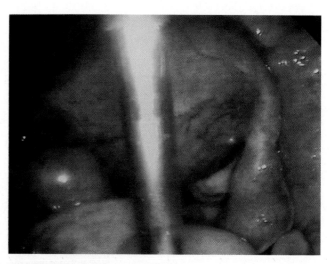

FIGURE 12.3 "Retort" tube of PID.

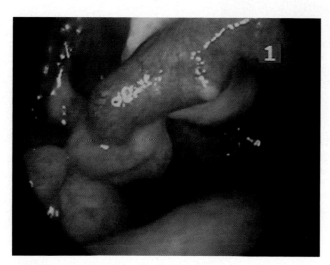

FIGURE 12.2 Pyosalpinx and blunted fimbria associated with acute PID.

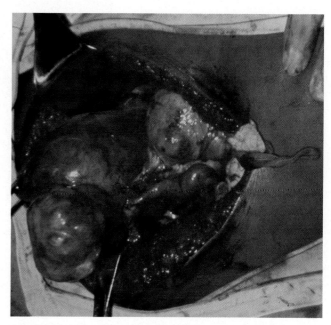

FIGURE 12.4 Pyosalpinx ("retort" tube).

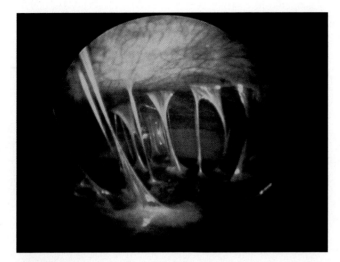

FIGURE 12.5 Fitz-Hugh and Curtis syndrome.

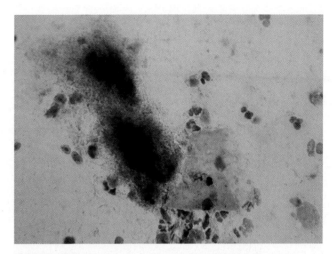

FIGURE 12.7 Pap smear demonstrating *Actinomyces*.

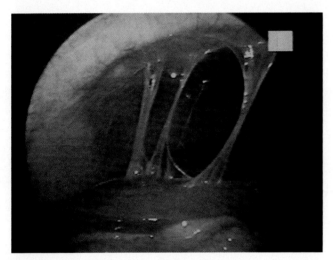

FIGURE 12.6 "Banjo-string" adhesions of Fitz-Hugh and Curtis syndrome.

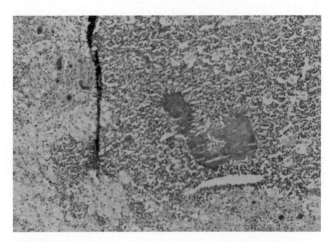

FIGURE 12.8 Sulfur granule *Actinomyces* of endometrium.

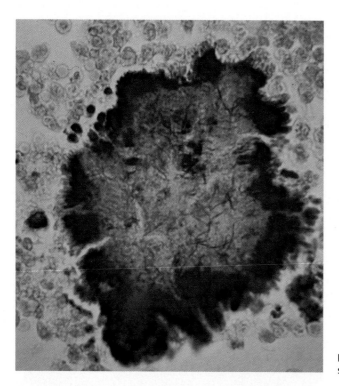

FIGURE 12.9 Sulfur granules of *Actinomyces israeli*. 400 × Gram stain.

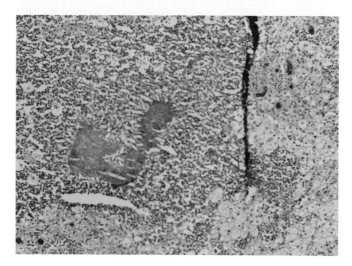

FIGURE 12.10 Sulfur granules of *Actinomyces* in wall of tuboovarian abscess.

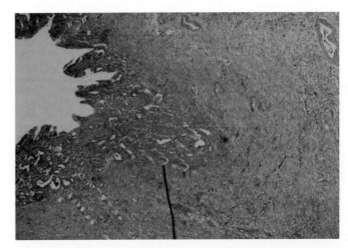

FIGURE 12.11 H&E stain *Actinomyces* of endometrium low power.

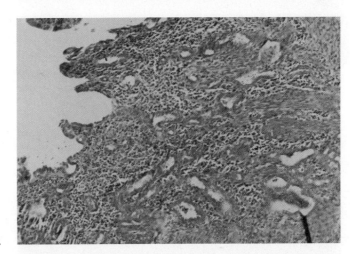

FIGURE 12.12 H&E stain *Actinomyces* of endometrium.

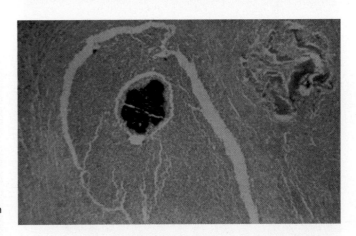

FIGURE 12.13 Gram stain of sulfur granules of *Actinomyces* in the endometrium.

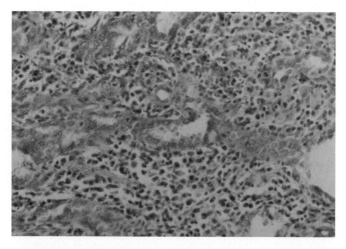

FIGURE 12.14 *Actinomyces* infection of the endometrium 400×.

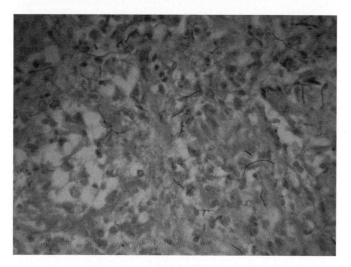

FIGURE 12.15 *Actinomyces israeli* in wall of tuboovarian abscess.

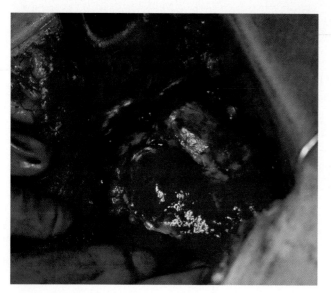

FIGURE 12.16 Tuboovarian abscess at exploratory laparotomy.

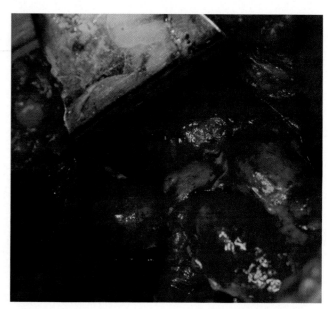

FIGURE 12.17 Tuboovarian abscess at exploratory laparotomy.

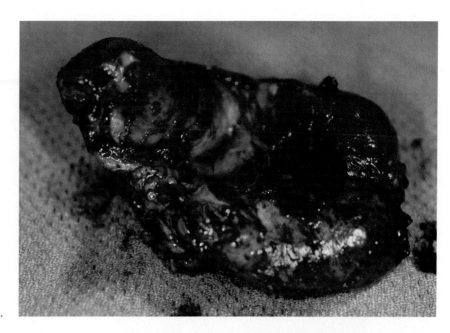

FIGURE 12.18 Tuboovarian abscess.

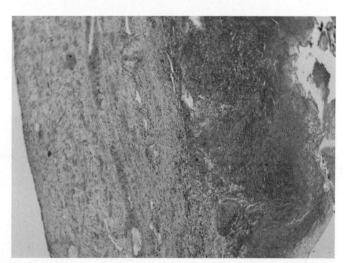

FIGURE 12.19 Wall of tuboovarian abscess.

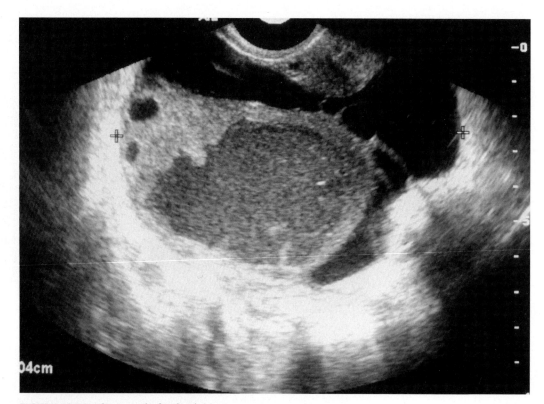

FIGURE 12.20 Ultrasound of polysalpinx.

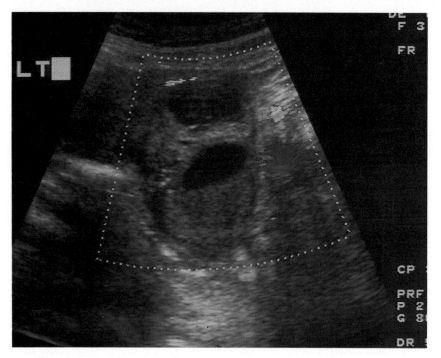

FIGURE 12.21 Doppler ultrasound of tuboovarian abscess.

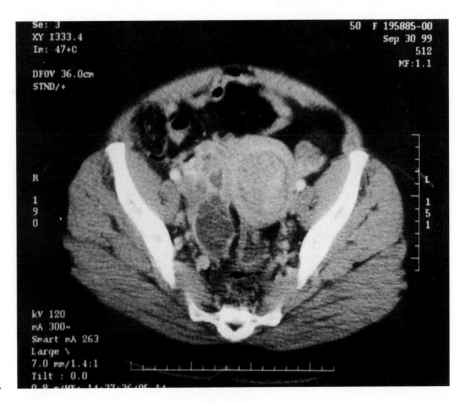

FIGURE 12.22 MRI of tuboovarian abscess.

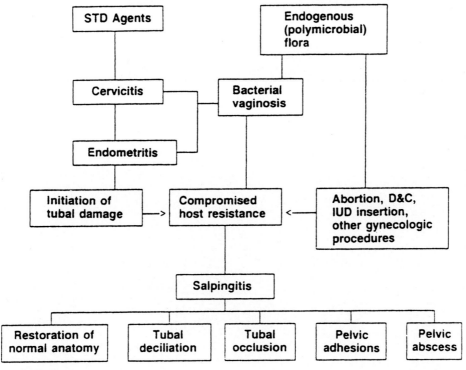

FIGURE 12.23 Possible interrelation of sexually transmitted organisms and endogenous organisms in the pathogenesis of PID.

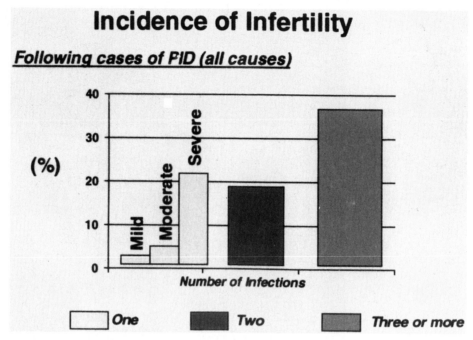

FIGURE 12.24 Incidence of infertility after cases of PID: number of episodes and severity of fallopian tube disease at laparoscopy.

BOX 12.1

Recommended Regimens for Oral Treatment of Acute Pelvic Inflammatory Disease

Regimen A
- Ofloxacin 400 mg PO b.i.d. for 14 days or Levofloxacin 500 mg PO q.d.
  plus
- Metronidazole 500 mg PO b.i.d. for 14 days

Regimen B
- Ceftriaxone 250 mg IM in a single dose
  or
- Cefoxitin 2 g IM plus probenecid 1 g PO in a single dose concurrently
  or
- Other parenteral third-generation cephalosporin (e.g., ceftizoxime or cefotaxime)
  plus
- Doxycycline 100 mg PO b.i.d. for 14 days with or without metronidabole 500 mg PO b.i.d. for 14 days

Note: From Centers for Disease Control and Prevention. Sexually transmitted diseases treatment guidelines *MMWR* 2002;51(No. RR-6):1–78, with permission.

BOX 12.2

Recommended Regimens for Parenteral (Inpatient or Outpatient) Treatment of Acute Pelvic Inflammatory Disease

Regimen A
- Cefotetan 2 g IV every 12 hours
  or
- Cefoxitin 2 g IV every 6 hours
  plus
- Doxycycline 100 mg IV or PO every 12 hours
  (Regimen given for at least 24 hours after patient clinically improves.[a] After discharge from hospital, continue doxycycline 100 mg PO b.i.d. for 14 days.)

Regimen B
- Clindamycin 900 mg IV every 8 hours
  plus
- Gentamicin loading dose IV or IM (2 mg/kg) followed by maintenance dose (1.5 mg/kg) every 8 hours
  (Regimen given for at least 24 hours after the patient improves.[a] After discharge from the hospital, continue doxycycline 100 mg PO b.i.d. for 14 days or clindamycin 450 mg PO q.i.d. to complete 14 days of therapy.)

[a] Most trials have used parenteral treatment for at least 48 hours after patient demonstrates clinical improvement.
Note: From Centers for Disease Control and Prevention. Sexually transmitted diseases treatment guidelines *MMWR* 2002;51(No. RR-6):1–78, with permission.

13

URINARY TRACT INFECTION

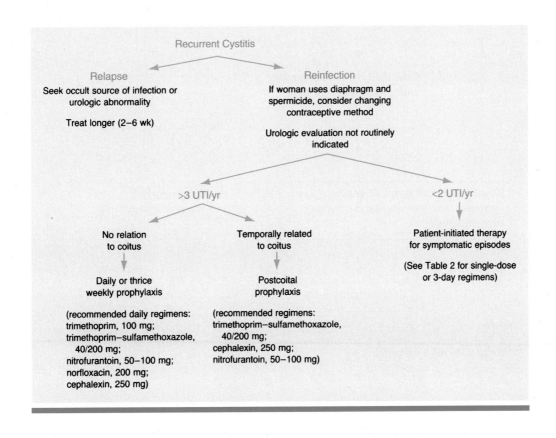

Recurrent Cystitis

Relapse

Seek occult source of infection or
urologic abnormality

Treat longer (2–6 wk)

Reinfection

If woman uses diaphragm and
spermicide, consider changing
contraceptive method

Urologic evaluation not routinely
indicated

>3 UTI/yr

<2 UTI/yr

No relation
to coitus

Temporally related
to coitus

Patient-initiated therapy
for symptomatic episodes

(See Table 2 for single-dose
or 3-day regimens)

Daily or thrice
weekly prophylaxis

Postcoital
prophylaxis

(recommended daily regimens:
trimethoprim, 100 mg;
trimethoprim–sulfamethoxazole,
    40/200 mg;
nitrofurantoin, 50–100 mg;
norfloxacin, 200 mg;
cephalexin, 250 mg)

(recommended regimens:
trimethoprim–sulfamethoxazole,
    40/200 mg;
cephalexin, 250 mg;
nitrofurantoin, 50–100 mg)

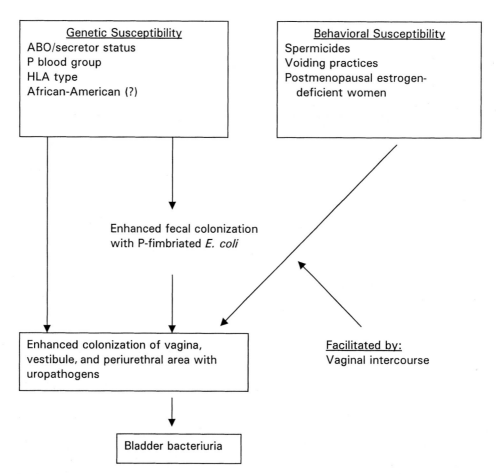

FIGURE 13.1 Host Factors in the pathogenesis of urinary tract infections in women. (From Sobel JD. Pathogenesis of urinary tract infection: role of host defenses. *Infect Dis Clin North Am* 1997;11:531–549, with permission.)

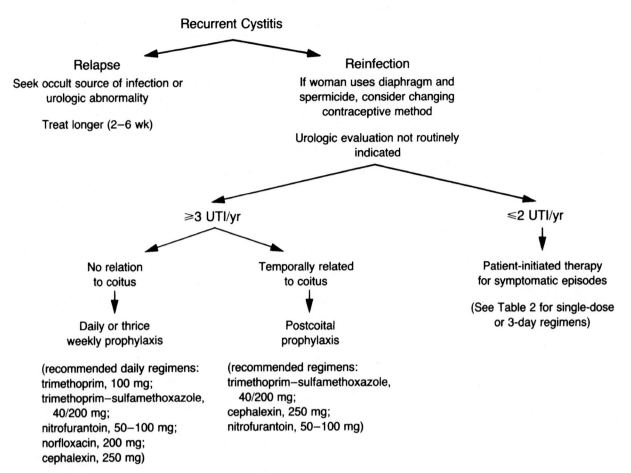

FIGURE 13.2 Strategies for managing recurrent cystitis in women.

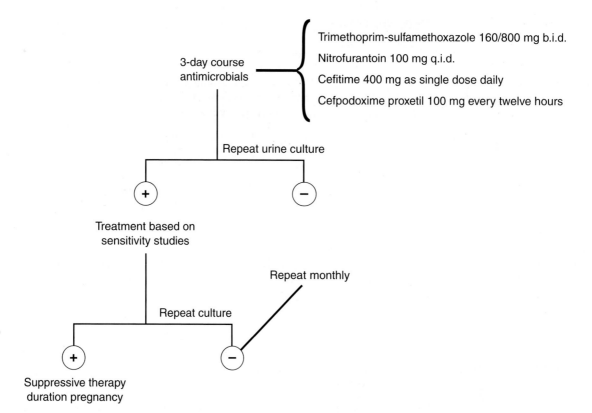

FIGURE 13.3 Management plan for asymptomatic bacteriuria in pregnancy.

BOX 13.1

Recommended 3-Day Regimens for Acute Uncomplicated Cystitis in Young Women

Trimethoprim-sulfamethoxazole 160/800 mg every
    12 hours
Trimethoprim 100 mg every 12 hours
Quinolones

- Ciprofloxacin 250 mg q12h
- Enoxacin 400 mg q12h
- Lomefloxacin 400 mg q24h
- Ofloxacin 200 mg q12h
- Norfloxacin 400 mg q12h
- Fleroxacin

BOX 13.2

Recommended Regimens for Acute Uncomplicated Pyelonephritis in Nonpregnant Young Women

Oral (10–14 days)

- Trimethoprim-sulfamethoxazole 160/800 mg every
  12 hours
- Ciprofloxacin 500 mg every 12 hours
- Ofloxacin 200–300 mg every 12 hours
- Norfloxacin 400 mg every 12 hours
- Lomefloxacin 400 mg every 24 hours
- Eroxcin 400 mg
- Levofloxacin 250 mg q.d.
- Sparfloxacin 400 mg day 1, then 200 mg q.d.
- Cefixime 400 mg q.d.
- Cefpodoxime proxetil 200 mg every 12 hours

Parenteral[a]

- Trimethoprim-sulfamethoxazole 160/800 mg
- Ceftriaxone 1–2 g every 24 hours
- Ciprofloxacin 200–400 mg
- Ofloxacin 200–400 mg
- Gentamicin 3–5 mg/kg single dose every day or
  1 mg/kg every 8 hours ± ampicillin 1 g every 6 hours
- Levofloxacin 250 mg every 24 hours

---

[a]Followed by oral antibiotics after clinical response to complete
10–14-day course.

14

PERINATAL INFECTIONS

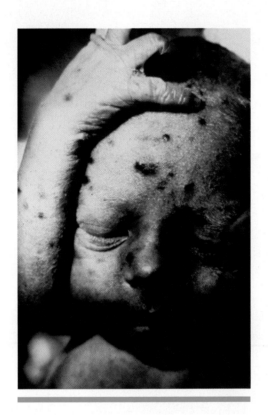

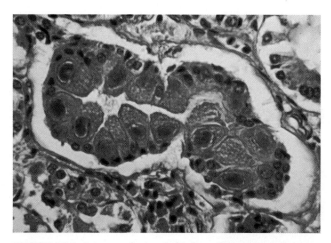

FIGURE 14.1 Cytomegalovirus infection. Characteristic intranuclear inclusions are seen in cells of the glomerulus.

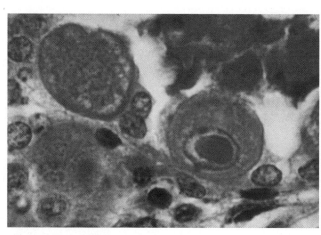

FIGURE 14.2 Cytomegalovirus infection. A close up view of intranuclear inclusions in renal cells.

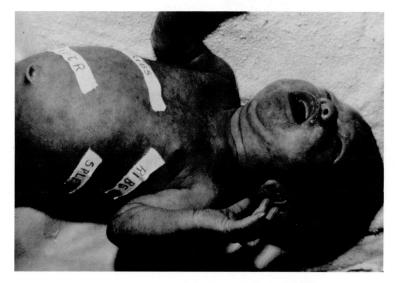

FIGURE 14.3 Congenital CMV infection with hepatosplenomegaly.

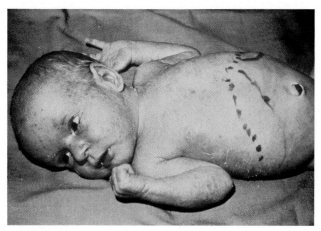

FIGURE 14.4 An infant with congenital cytomegalovirus infection. Infant had jaundice, hepatosplenomegaly, and petechiae.

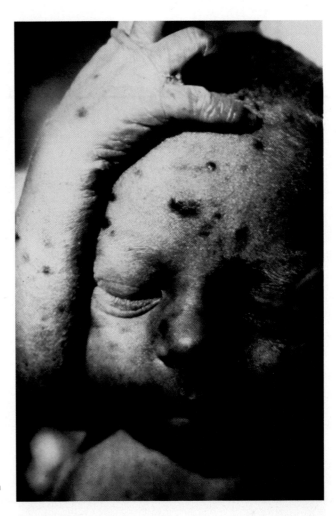

FIGURE 14.5 Congenital CMV "blueberry muffin" baby with jaundice and thrombocytopenia purpura.

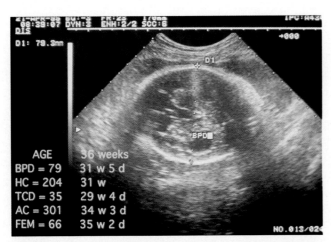

FIGURE 14.6 Cytomegalovirus infection. Head ultrasound showing a small biparietal diameter and a small transcerebellar diameter plus intranuclear calcifications.

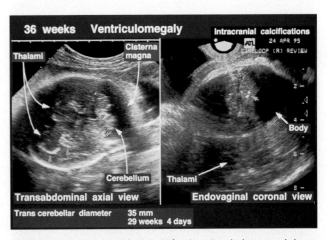

FIGURE 14.7 Cytomegalovirus infection: Fetal ultrasound showing intracranial calcification.

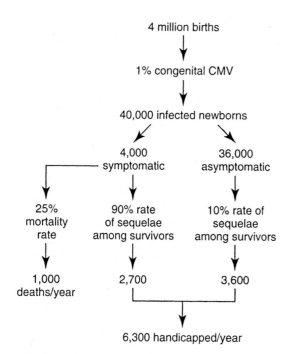

4 million births

↓

1% congenital CMV

↓

40,000 infected newborns

↙ ↘

4,000 symptomatic   36,000 asymptomatic

↓ (25% mortality rate)   ↓ (90% rate of sequelae among survivors)   ↓ (10% rate of sequelae among survivors)

1,000 deaths/year   2,700   3,600

↓

6,300 handicapped/year

FIGURE 14.8 Public health impact of congenital cytomegalovirus (CMV) infection in the United States.

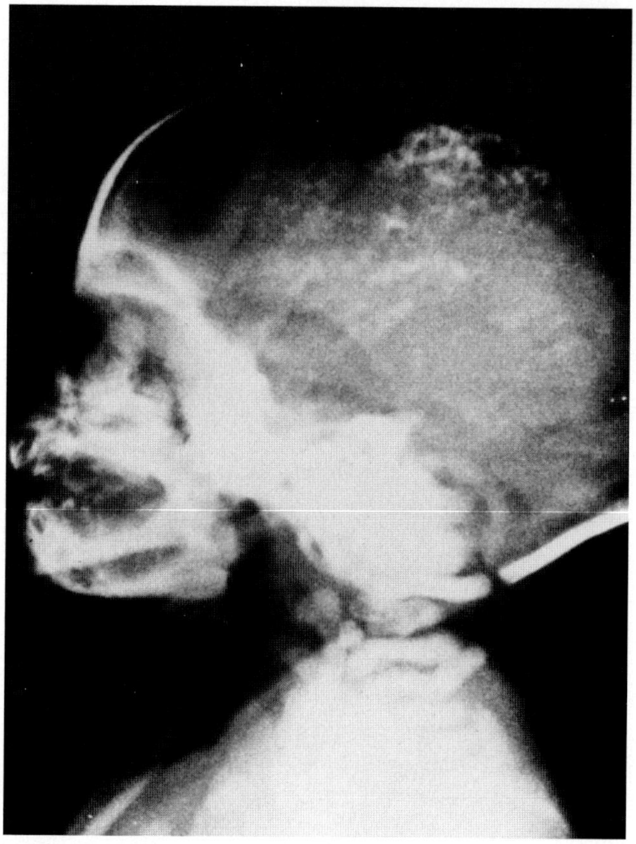

FIGURE 14.10 Periventricular calcifications in congenital CMV lateral skull x-ray.

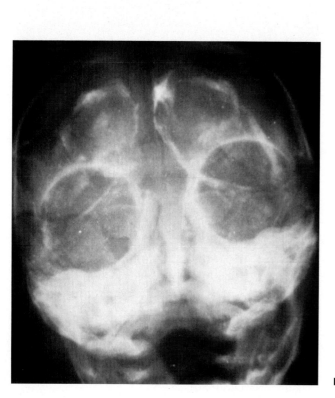

FIGURE 14.9 Periventricular calcifications of congenital CMV.

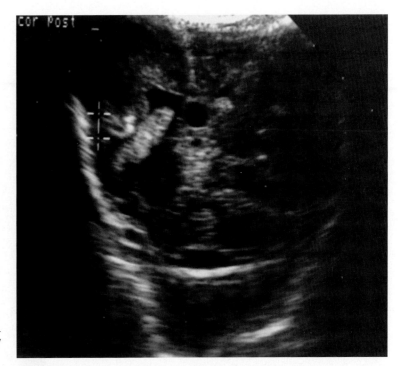

FIGURE 14.11 Neonatal brain scan revealing right-sided periventricular calcification in congenital CMV infection.

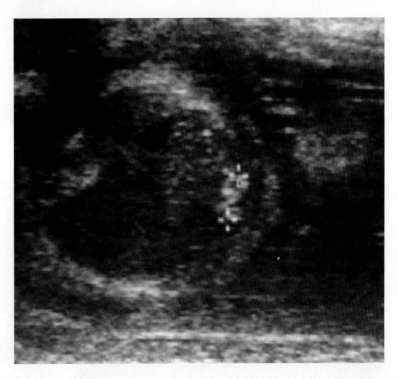

FIGURE 14.12 Ultrasound of 22 weeks' gestation with calcification within fetal liver.

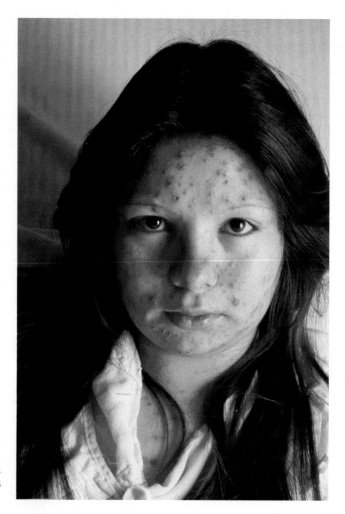

FIGURE 14.13 Varicella infection. A pregnant patient with chickenpox during the first trimester. Characteristic healing pox lesions are abundant on the face.

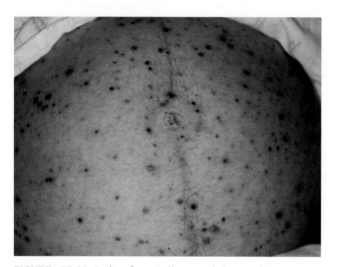

FIGURE 14.14 Rash of varicella on abdomen in pregnant woman.

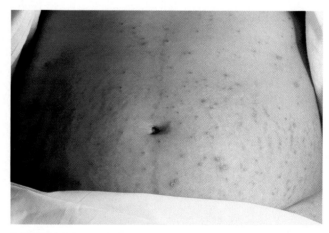

FIGURE 14.15 Varicella in pregnancy showing healing lesions on the abdomen.

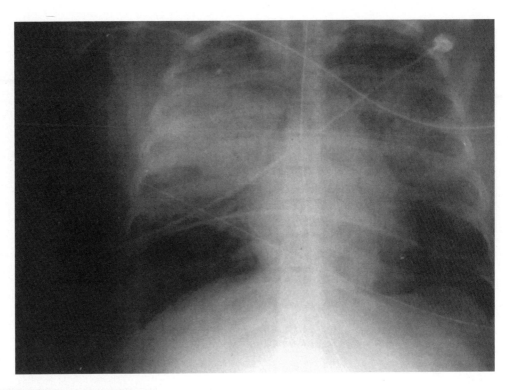

FIGURE 14.16 Varicella infection with pneumonia.

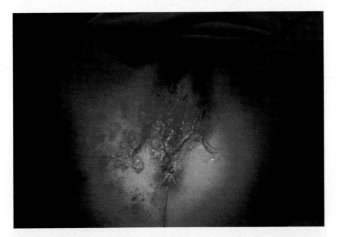

FIGURE 14.17 Severe lumbosacral (perineal) shingles in an immunosuppressed patient after bone marrow transplant.

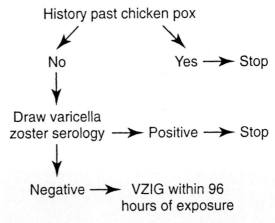

FIGURE 14.18 Protocol for management of pregnant women exposed to varicella.

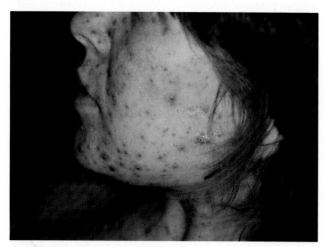

FIGURE 14.19 Rash of varicella: Crops of lesions in various stages (vesicles, pustules, scabs).

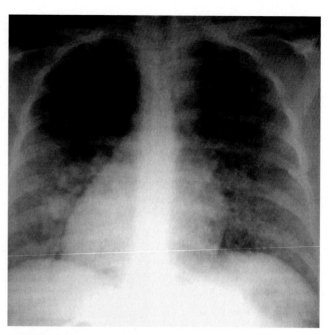

FIGURE 14.21 Varicella pneumonia.

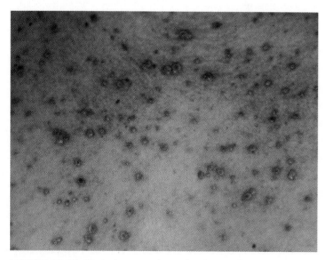

FIGURE 14.20 Vesicular-pustular rash of varicella: close-up.

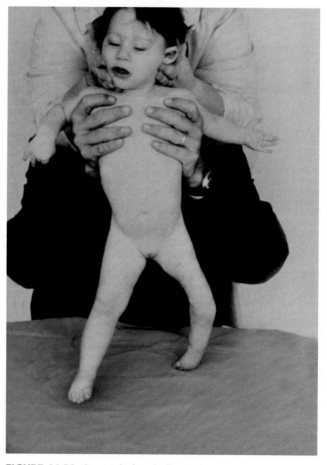

FIGURE 14.22 Congenital varicella syndrome.

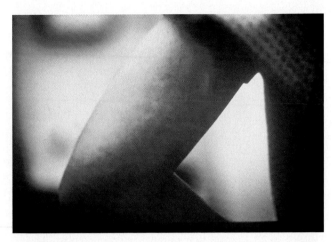

FIGURE 14.23 Parvovirus infection. Photograph demonstrates the lacelike reticulated rash on the arm of a youngster with fifth disease.

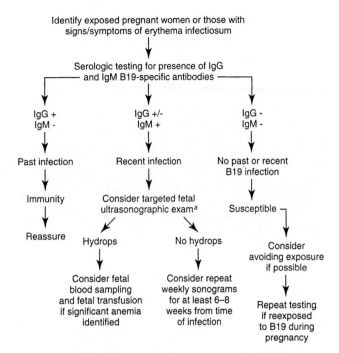

Identify exposed pregnant women or those with signs/symptoms of erythema infectiosum

Serologic testing for presence of IgG and IgM B19-specific antibodies

IgG +, IgM − → Past infection → Immunity → Reassure

IgG +/−, IgM + → Recent infection → Consider targeted fetal ultrasonographic exam[a] → Hydrops → Consider fetal blood sampling and fetal transfusion if significant anemia identified; No hydrops → Consider repeat weekly sonograms for at least 6–8 weeks from time of infection

IgG −, IgM − → No past or recent B19 infection → Susceptible → Consider avoiding exposure if possible → Repeat testing if reexposed to B19 during pregnancy

[a]Alternatively, MSAFP may be used as initial screening tool at weekly intervals. Elevated MSAFP indicates fetus requiring serial sonography to assess for presence of hydrops.

FIGURE 14.25 Suggested protocol for management of pregnant women exposed to parvovirus B19.

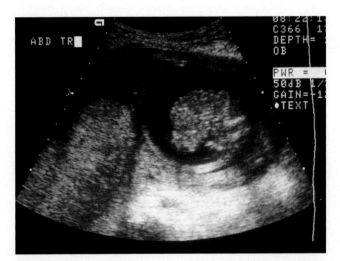

FIGURE 14.24 Parvovirus infection. Ultrasound showing ascites in a fetus with hydrops.

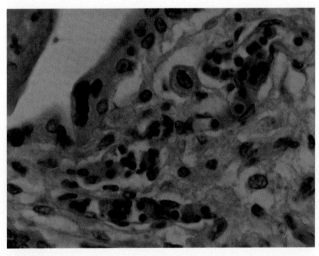

FIGURE 14.26 Human Parvovirus B19 in red blood cells of placenta.

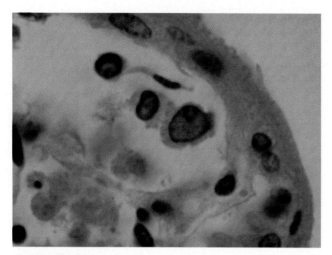

FIGURE 14.27 Human Parvovirus B19 in placenta.

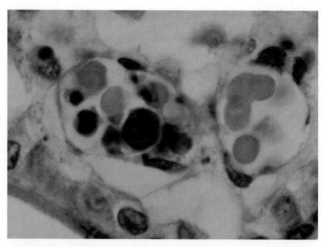

FIGURE 14.28 Human Parvovirus B19 infection in placenta.

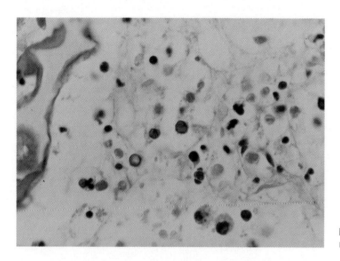

FIGURE 14.29 Human Parvovirus B19 infection in fetal bone marrow.

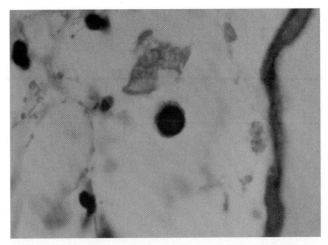

FIGURE 14.30 Human Parvovirus B19 in fetal bone marrow.

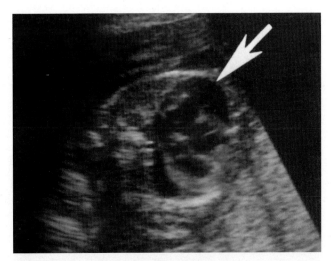

FIGURE 14.32 Ultrasound demonstrating pericardial effusion at 23 weeks' age gestation with Parvovirus infection.

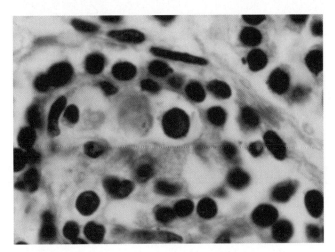

FIGURE 14.31 Human Parvovirus B19 in fetal kidney.

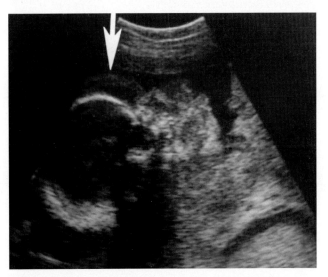

FIGURE 14.33 Scalp edema in fetal Parvovirus infection.

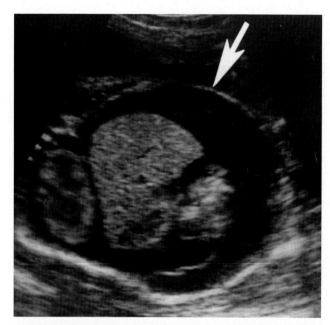

FIGURE 14.34 Ultrasound demonstrating fetal ascites in Parvovirus infection.

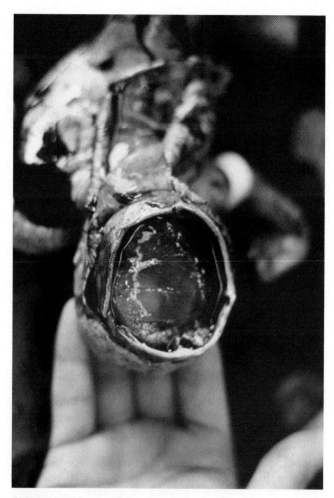

FIGURE 14.35 Toxoplasmosis.

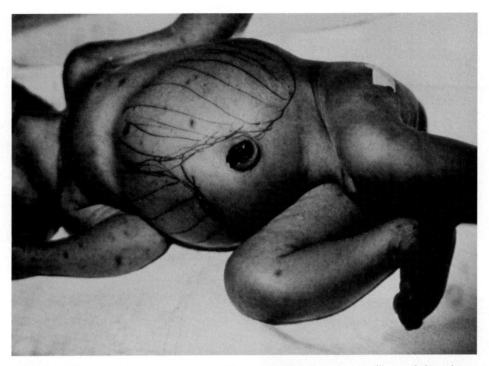

FIGURE 14.36 Congenital toxoplasmosis with hepatosplenomegaly, jaundice, and thrombocy-topenia purpura.

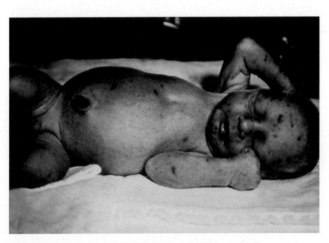

FIGURE 14.37 Congenital Rubella infection at birth.

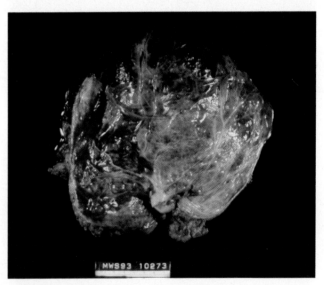

FIGURE 14.38 Listeriosis infection of placenta.

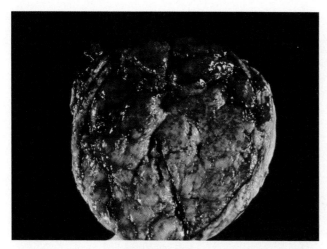

FIGURE 14.39 Listeriosis infection of placenta.

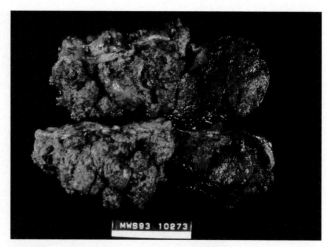

FIGURE 14.40 Cross-section of placenta infected with listeriosis.

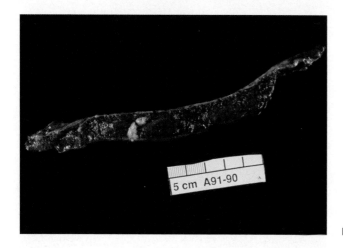

FIGURE 14.41 Placenta with listeriosis.

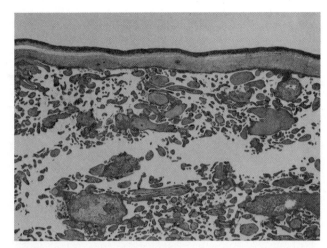

FIGURE 14.42 Listeriosis of placenta.

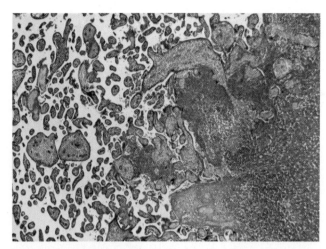

FIGURE 14.44 Placental abscess resulting from listeriosis.

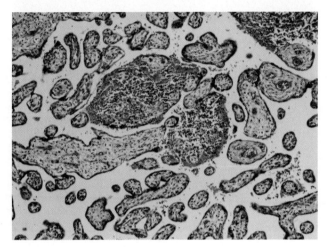

FIGURE 14.43 Listeriosis infection of Chorionic villi.

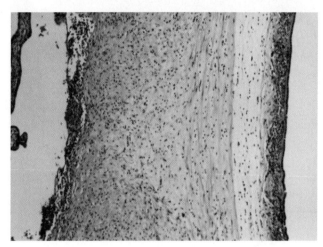

FIGURE 14.45 Microabscesses of listeriosis in placenta.

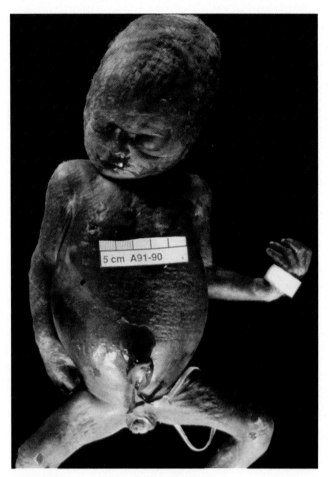

FIGURE 14.46 Stillbirth with listeriosis.

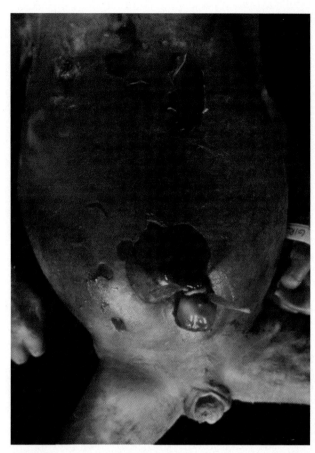

FIGURE 14.47 Stillbirth with listeriosis.

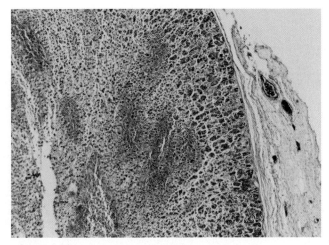

FIGURE 14.48 Listeriosis: fetal adrenal.

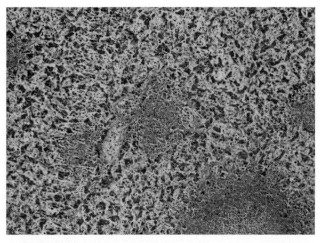

FIGURE 14.50 Listeriosis: fetal liver.

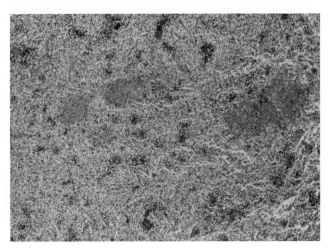

FIGURE 14.49 Listeriosis: fetal spleen.

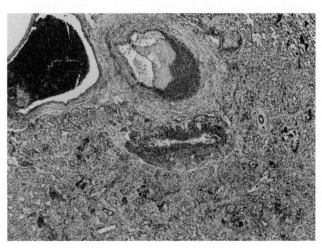

FIGURE 14.51 Listeriosis: fetal lung.

15

PREMATURE RUPTURE OF
THE MEMBRANES

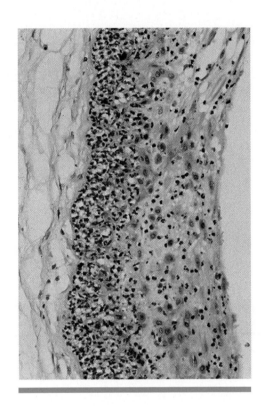

BOX 15.1

**Summary of Management:
PROM <24 Weeks**

- Induction versus expectancy, depending on gestational age and patient desires
- No data on steroids, tocolytics, or antibiotics (for GBS prophylaxis or prolonging pregnancy)

BOX 15.3

**Summary of Management:
PROM at 33–35 Weeks**

- Expectancy versus induction, especially if "mature"
- GBS prophylaxis

BOX 15.2

**Summary of Management:
PROM at 25–32 Weeks**

- Expectancy
- GBS prophylaxis
- Corticosteroids
- Antibiotics for 7 days (ampicillin + erythromycin *or* clindamycin) or alternative regimens
- ??Tocolytics for 48 hours

BOX 15.4

**Summary of Management:
PROM at or Near Term**

- Induction usually preferred, with oxytocin or prostaglandin preparations (especially with unripe cervix)
- GBS prophylaxis with ROM >12–18 hours

16

INTRAAMNIOTIC INFECTION

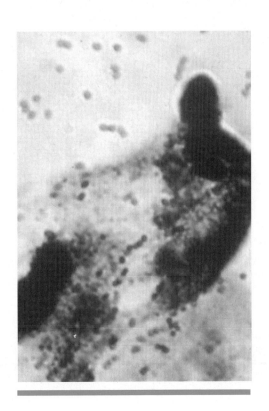

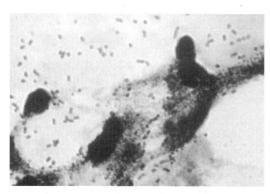

FIGURE 16.1 Gram stain of amniotic fluid from a patient with clinical intraamniotic infection due to group B streptococci. Note numerous Gram-positive cocci.

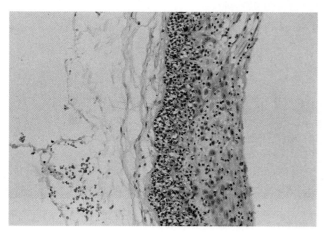

FIGURE 16.2 Histologic chorioamnionitis. Note the intense polymorphonuclear infiltrate in the membranes.

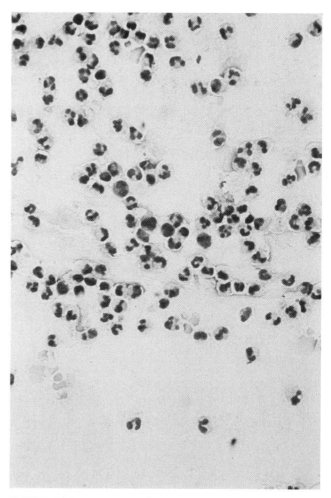

FIGURE 16.3 Gram stain of purulent amnionic fluid showing extensive numbers of polymorphonuclear leukocytes.

TABLE 16.1 AMNIOTIC FLUID ISOLATES IN 404 CASES OF INTRAAMNIOTIC INFECTION

Organism[a]	No. (%)
Group B streptococci	59 (14.6)
Escherichia coli	33 (8.2)
Enterococci	22 (5.4)
Gardnerella vaginalis	99 (24.5)
Peptostreptococci	38 (9.4)
Bacteroides bivius	119 (29.4)
Bacteroides fragilis	14 (3.4)
Fusobacterium sp	22 (5.4)
Mycoplasma hominis	123 (30.4)
Ureaplasma urealyticum	190 (47.0)

[a] For bacteria, all isolates shown were found in concentrations $>10^2$ CFU/mL. Genital mycoplasmas were cultured qualitatively.
Note: From Sperling RS, Newton E, Gibbs RS. Intraaminiotic infection in low-birth-weight infants. *J Infect Dis* 1988;157:113, with permission.

BOX 16.1

Clinical Measures to Prevent Chorioamnionitis

- Identify dystocia promptly and treat hypotonic dysfunctional labor promptly with oxytocin.
- In patients with PROM at term, induce labor with either oxytocin or prostaglandin preparations.
- In patients with preterm PROM and without contractions, give broad-spectrum antibiotics such as ampicillin-amoxicillin plus erythromycin for 7 days.
- Follow CDC/ACOG guidelines for prevention of perinatal GBS infection.
- For patients with preterm labor but without rupture of membranes, perinatal GBS guidelines should be followed, but broad-spectrum antibiotics given to prevent chorioamnionitis have not been effective.

17

SUBCLINICAL INFECTION AS A CAUSE OF PREMATURE LABOR

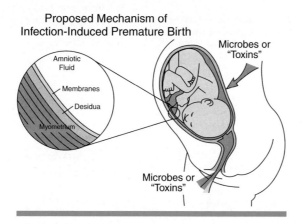

Proposed Mechanism of
Infection-Induced Premature Birth

Amniotic
Fluid

Membranes

Desidua

Myometrium

Microbes or
"Toxins"

Microbes or
"Toxins"

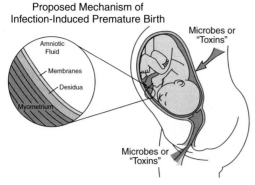

Proposed Mechanism of
Infection-Induced Premature Birth

FIGURE 17.1 Proposed mechanism of infection-induced premature birth. Microbes or microbial toxins enter the uterine cavity by an ascending or bloodborne route. An interaction then occurs, most likely in the decidua, to release cytokines and prostaglandins.

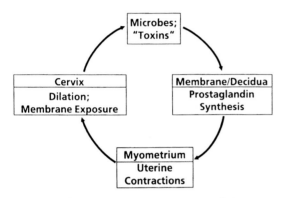

FIGURE 17.2 Diagrammatic representation of the proposed links between infection and preterm uterine contractions.

BOX 17.1

Evidence for Subclinical Infection as a Cause of Preterm Birth (PTB)

1. Histologic chorioamnionitis is increased in PTB
2. Clinical infection is increased after PTB
3. There are significant associations of some lower genital tract organisms/infections with PTB or preterm premature rupture of the membranes
4. There are positive cultures of amniotic fluid or membranes from some patients with preterm labor/PTB
5. There are markers of infection in PTB
6. Bacteria or their products induce PTB in animal models
7. Some antibiotic trials have shown a lower rate of PTB or have deferred PTB

BOX 17.2

Use of Antibiotics During Prenatal Care to Prevent PTB

- Treat bacteriuria
- Treat *N. gonorrhoeae*
- Treat *C. trachomatis*
- Treat BV in high-risk patients (defined, for example, as those with previous preterm birth or previous preterm PROM) with an oral regimen for at least 7 drop.
- Do not treat *U. urealyticum* or GBS genital colonization

> **BOX 17.3**
>
> **Use of Antibiotics in Preterm Labor with Intact Membranes to Prevent PTB**
>
> - Do not give antibiotics routinely to prevent PTB.[a]
> - Although not standard, it may be reasonable to treat BV. Optimal dose and duration are not established.
>
> ---
> [a] GBS prophylaxis is indicated.

> **BOX 17.4**
>
> **Use of Antibiotics with PROM to Prevent PTB**
>
> - At 24–32 weeks, give broad-spectrum antibiotics such as ampicillin plus erythromycin for 7 days.
> - Other regimens also may be effective.
>
> ---
> [a] GBS prophylaxis should be indicated.

18

POSTPARTUM INFECTION

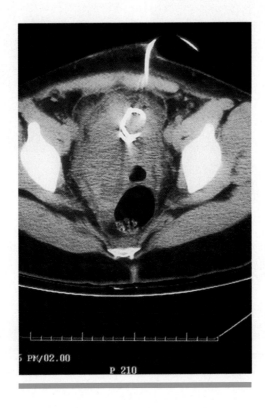

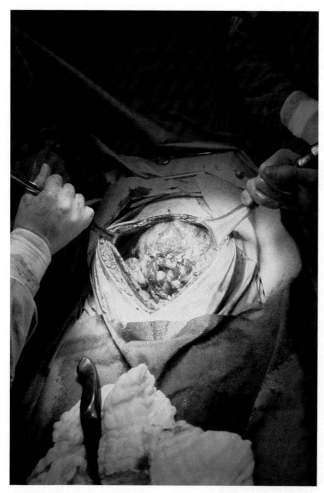

FIGURE 18.1 Laparotomy in a case of Group A Streptococcal sepsis over 25 ml of purulent peritoneal fluid was drained and hysterectomy was necessary.

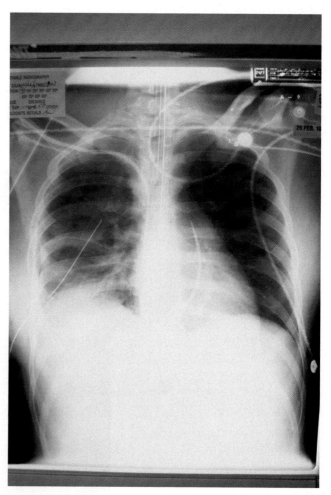

FIGURE 18.2 Chest x-ray from a patient with Group A Streptococcal sepsis and adult respiratory distress syndrome.

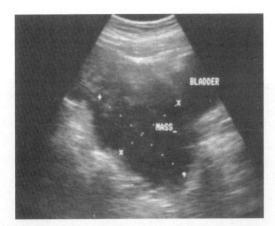

FIGURE 18.3 Longitudinal scan demonstrating an 8 x 5-cm mass lateral to the uterus in a patient with persistent fever after vaginal delivery.

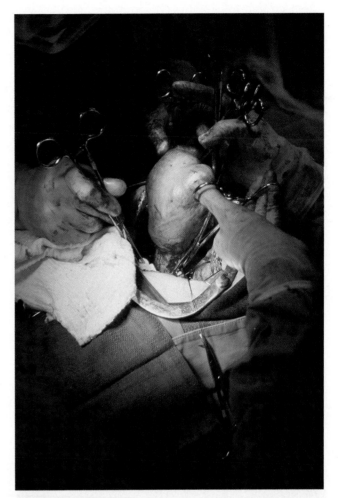

FIGURE 18.5 Laparotomy in a case of Clostridial myonecrosis.

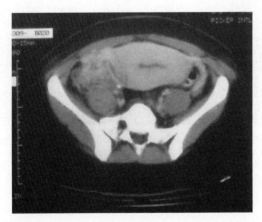

FIGURE 18.4 Computerized tomographic scan in a patient with persistent fever after cesarean delivery. Note the asymmetric "moth-eaten" mass adjacent to uterus (on **left** in scan) and anterior to the psoas muscle. This was consistent with an infected hematoma.

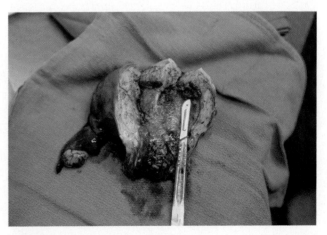

FIGURE 18.6 Hysterectomy specimen from a case of Clostridial myonecrosis. Note the black necrotic tissue in the uterine cavity and over the lower uterine segment.

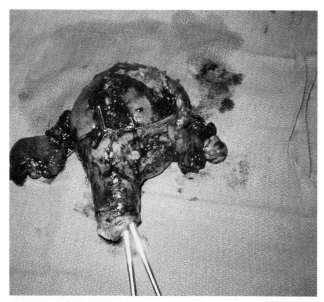

FIGURE 18.7 Infected uterus with necrosis of uterine incision after cesarean delivery.

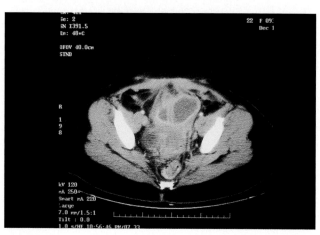

FIGURE 18.9 Parauterine abscess in a patient after cesarean delivery.

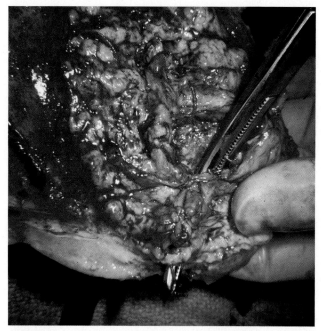

FIGURE 18.8 Close up of necrosis showing breakdown of uterine incision.

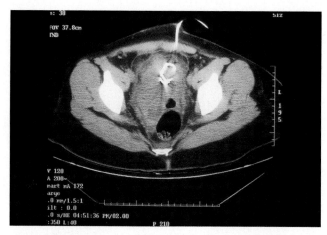

FIGURE 18.10 Computerized tomographic scan showing percutaneous placement of a pigtail catheter in an abscess after cesarean section (same case as shown in previous figure).

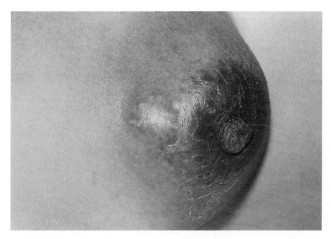

FIGURE 18.11 Mastitis.

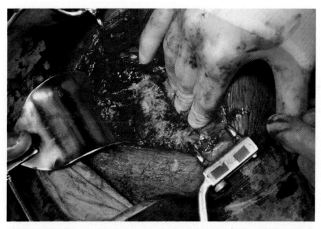

FIGURE 18.13 Postcesarean delivery abscess. Laparotomy in the case in Figure 18.12. Hysterectomy was necessary.

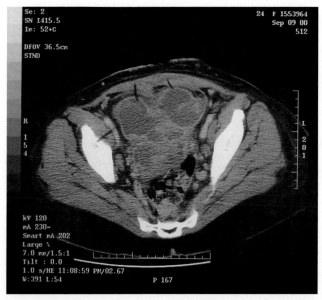

FIGURE 18.12 Postcesarean delivery abscess. CT scan showing multiloculated abscesses anteriorly and low in the pelvis in the region of uterine incision.

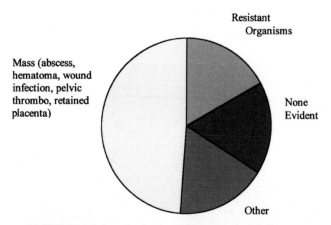

FIGURE 18.14 Causes of poor response to antibiotics.

Postpartum endometritis

Initial treatment with broad-spectrum regimen, intravenously

Resolution, usually within 48–72 hours
- Discontinue IV antibiotics after patient has been afebrile and free of signs of infection for 24–48 hours
- No oral antibiotics needed, except under special circumstances (such as bacteremia)

Persistent signs and symptoms of infection
- Interim history and physical examination to rule out other sources of infection
- Review culture results for resistant organism(s)
- Imaging studies to identify pelvic mass
- Consider antibiotic level as for gentamicin

Consider:
- Change in antibiotic dose
- Change in antibiotic regimen, based upon confirmed or suspected organisms
- Drain abscess or hematoma
- If septic thrombophlebitis, continuing antibiotics usually suffices anticoagulation or excision of thrombosed vessel(s) in special circumstances

FIGURE 18.15 Algorithm for treating postpartum endometritis.

TABLE 18.1 ENDOMETRIAL ISOLATES (COLLECTED BY A TRIPLE-LUMEN CATHETER) FROM 51 PATIENTS WITH POSTPARTUM ENDOMETRITIS

Isolate(s)	No. (%) of Isolates
Facultative Gram-positive	51 (40)
Group B streptococci	8 (6)
Enterococci	7 (5)
Staphylococcus epidermidis	9 (7)
Lactobacilli	4 (3)
Diphtheroids	2 (2)
Staphylococcus aureus	1 (1)
Facultative Gram-negative	28 (22)
Gardnerella vaginalis	15 (22)
Escherichia coli	6 (5)
Enterobacter sp	2 (2)
Proteus mirabilis	2 (2)
Other	3 (2)
Anaerobes	49 (38)
Bacteroides bivius	11 (9)
Other *Bacteroides* sp	9 (7)
Peptococci-peptostreptococci	22 (17)
Mycoplasmas	
Ureaplasma urealyticum	39 (30)
Mycoplasma hominis	11 (9)
Chlamydial trachomatis	2 (2)

Note: From Rosene K, Eschenbach DA, Tompkins LS, et al. Polymicrobial early postpartum endometritis with facultative and anaerobic bacteria, genital mycoplasmas and *C. trachomatis*: treatment with piperacillin or cefoxitin. *J Infect Dis* 1986;153:1028, with permission.

TABLE 18.2 SELECTED REGIMENS FOR INITIAL PARENTERAL THERAPY OF POSTPARTUM ENDOMETRITIS

Regimen	Organisms "Resistant" to the Regimen	Comments
Clindamycin plus gentamicin	Mainly enterococci	Often a standard for comparison
Cefoxitin, cefotetan, or alternative cephalosporin-like antibiotics	Mainly enterococci	Avoid in cases of immediate hypersensitivity to penicillin
Ampicillin-sulbactam (Unasyn)		Contraindicated in cases of penicillin allergy
Ticarcillin-clavulanic acid (Timentin)	Some aerobic Gram-negative rods	
Piperacillin-tazobactam (Zosyn)	Some aerobic, Gram-negative rods,	
Piperacillin, mezlocillin, or other ureido penicillins	some *Staphylococcus aureus*	Contraindicated in cases of penicillin allergy
Clindamycin plus aztreonam	Mainly enterococci	Alternative to gentamicin plus clindamycin
Metronidazole plus gentamicin	Group B streptococci, enterococci, and other aerobic streptococci	Absence of streptococcal actively limits its role in endometritis
Imipenem/cilastatin, meropenem, and other carbapenems	Some clostridia, some *S. aureus*	Because of unusual spectrum of activity, reserve for treating difficult infections

19

WOUND AND EPISIOTOMY INFECTIONS

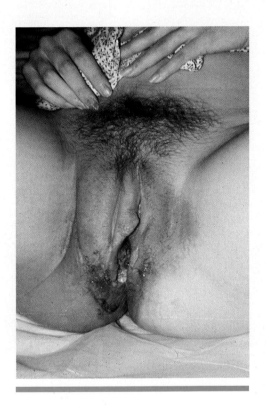

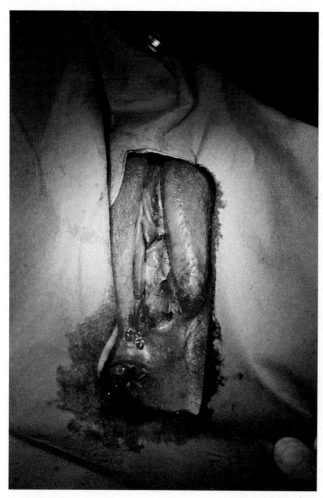

FIGURE 19.1 Preoperative photograph of patient with vulvar and perineal necrotizing fasciitis. Note asymmetric edema of labia majora and necrosis of left labia minora. Further debridement of necrotic tissue was necessary.

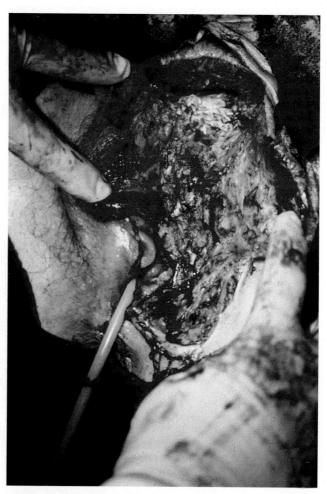

FIGURE 19.2 Intraoperative photograph of the case in Figure 19.1 of necrotizing fasciitis of the vulva. The catheter notes the location of the urethra. Note the extent of the dissection.

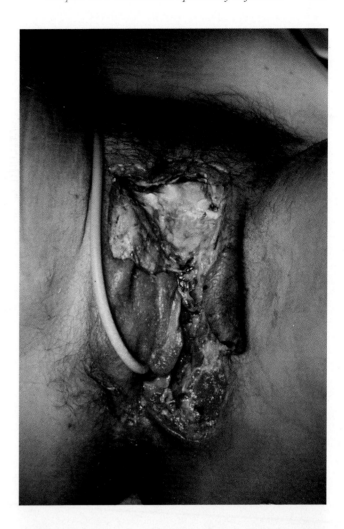

FIGURE 19.3 Second procedure of the case shown in Figure 19.1. Further debridement of devitalized tissue was necessary.

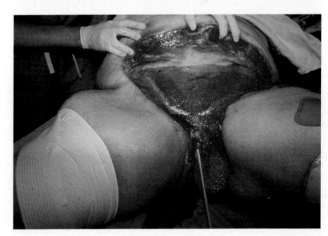

FIGURE 19.4 Extent of surgical excision in a diabetic with necrotizing fasciitis of the left vulva. Photograph taken on approximately hospital day 28, when closure was performed.

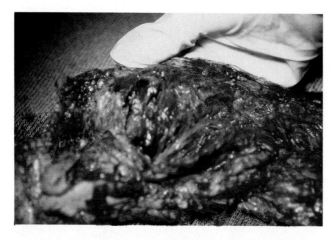

FIGURE 19.5 Gross specimen with necrotizing fasciitis. The skin is facing down. Note the black necrotic fascia.

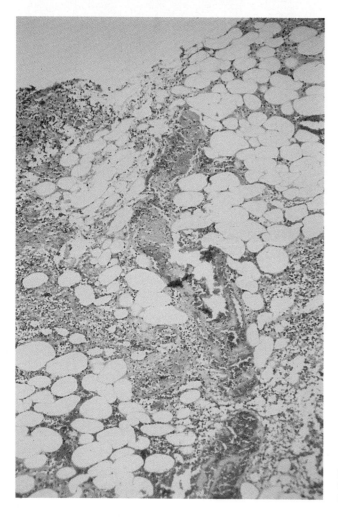

FIGURE 19.6 Microscopic appearance in a case of necrotizing fasciitis. Note the extent of necrosis with a degree of hemorrhage.

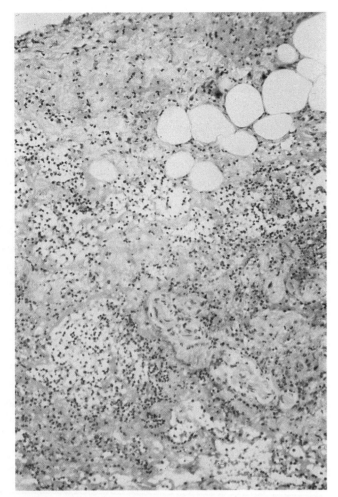

FIGURE 19.7 Microscopic appearance also of necrotizing fasciitis. Note the loss of architecture.

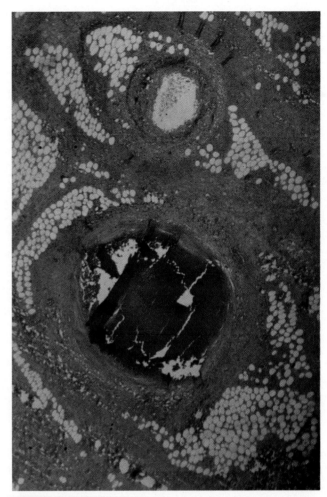

FIGURE 19.8 Microscopic section from a severe infection showing thrombosis.

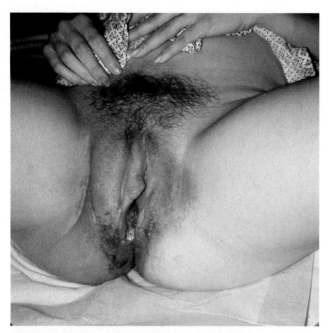

FIGURE 19.9 Puerperal necrotizing fasciitis of the right vulva following delivery and episiotomy. Note involvement of the buttocks, thighs, and mons. (From of Dr. James A. McGregor, University of Colorado Health Sciences Center, CO, USA, with permission.)

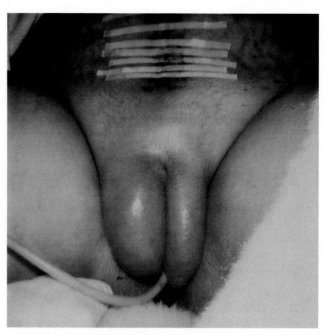

FIGURE 19.10 Vulvar edema of a noninfectious source. This patient had generalized edema from nephrotic syndrome with superimposed preeclampsia. Edema is bilateral and does not extend to the buttocks or abdominal wall.

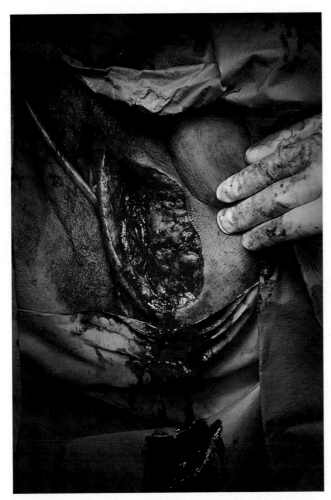

FIGURE 19.11 Incision and drainage of a vulvar abscess in a diabetic patient. No necrotizing fasciitis was noted.

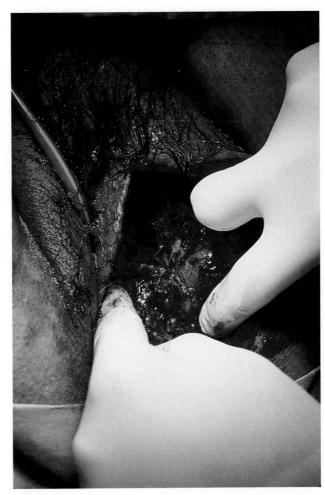

FIGURE 19.12 Close-up view of interior of vulvar abscess in case above.

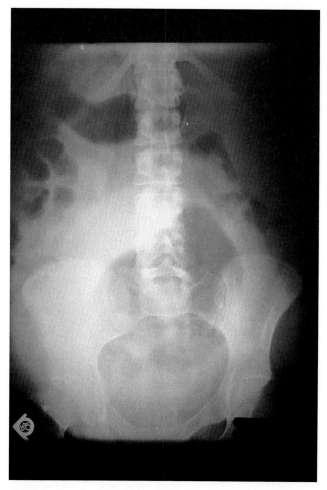

FIGURE 19.13 Radiograph showing large collection of gas.

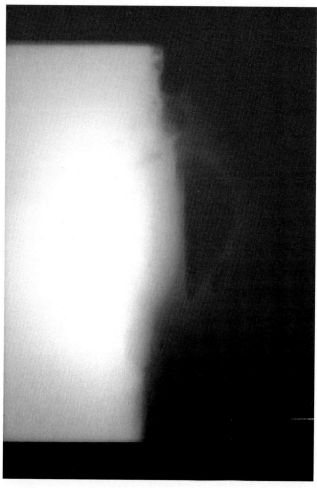

FIGURE 19.14 Lateral view from same case localizing the gas to the abdominal wall.

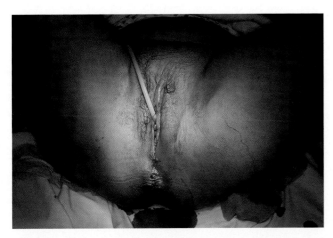

FIGURE 19.15 Extensive cellulitis of the mons, left labia, and left gluteal region in an immunocompromised woman on Imuran and Prednisone.

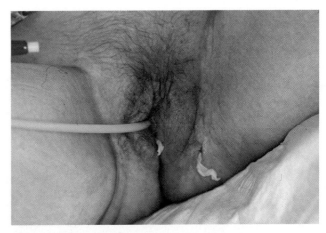

FIGURE 19.17 Photograph taken on postoperative day 1 in case in Figure 19.16. After exploration, with continued intravenous antibody therapy, there was marked resolution of the cellulitis within 24 hours.

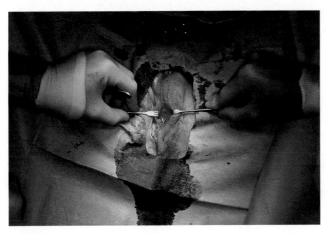

FIGURE 19.16 Surgical exploration of the case of cellulitis in Figure 19.15 to rule out necrotizing fasciitis. The fascia appeared healthy.

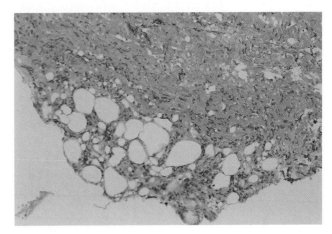

FIGURE 19.18 Histologic view of the case of cellulitis in Figure 19.15. Histologic examination showed only acute and chronic inflammation with some fat necrosis. This microscopic picture is also coming from the pathology resident.

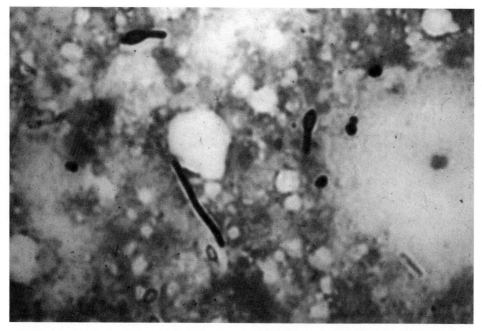

FIGURE 19.19 Gram-positive rods, some with spores, characteristic of *Clostridum perfringens*.

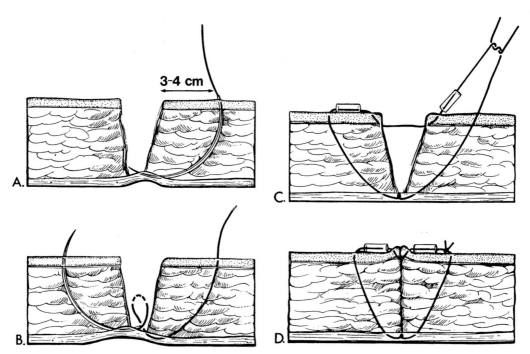

FIGURE 19.20 Technique of *en bloc* wound reclosure. **A:** The needle is passed from a point on the skin 3 cm to 4 cm from the wound edge through the superior part of the fascia at the wound base. **B:** The needle is withdrawn from the wound base, reintroduced into the fascia at the point from which it emerged with the first pass, and brought out through the skin at a point 3 cm to 4 cm from the opposite wound edge. **C:** Rubber suture guards are loaded onto the suture, the suture is brought across the incision incorporating the dermis and epidermis of the wound margins, and a second suture guard is loaded. **D:** The suture is tied, closing the wound. (From Walters MD, Dombroski RA, Davidson SA, et al. Reclosure of disrupted abdominal incisions. *Obstet Gynecol* 1990;76:597–602, with permission.)

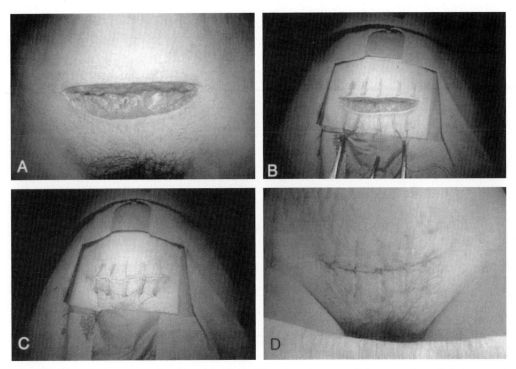

FIGURE 19.21 Walters' technique for closure. **A:** Wound at the start of the procedure. **B:** Sutures and rubber shods in place. **C:** Sutures are tied. Close of the procedure. **D:** Wound on postoperative (post-closure) day 10.

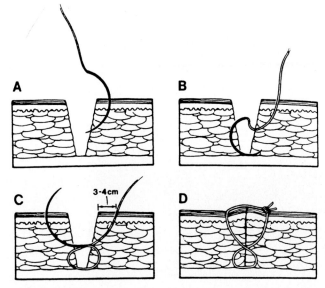

FIGURE 19.22 Technique of *en bloc* secondary closure. **A:** The needle is passed 3 cm to 4 cm from the edge of the incision to the base. **B, C:** Alternative technique if the incision is too deep for a single needle pass. **D:** The suture is tied, obliterating dead space and approximating the edges. (From Dadson MK, Magann EF, Meeks GR. A randomized comparison of secondary closure and secondary intention in patients with superficial wound dehiscence. *Obstet Gynecol* 1992;80:321–324, with permission.)

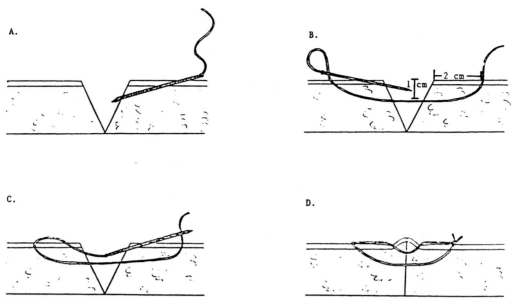

FIGURE 19.23 Superficial skin closure technique using vertical mattress sutures. (From Dodson, MK, Magann EF, Sullivan DL, et al. Extrafascial wound dehiscence: deep *en bloc* closure versus superficial skin closure. *Obstet Gynecol* 1994;83:142–145, with permission.)

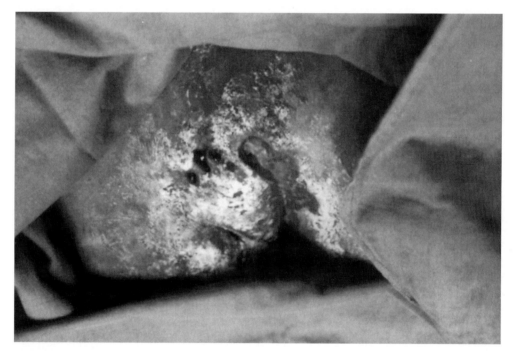

FIGURE 19.24 Progressive synergistic bacterial gangrene in a patient with stage IV carcinoma of the cervix. A central ulcerated area is seen in the left crural region and is surrounded by an irregular darker zone.

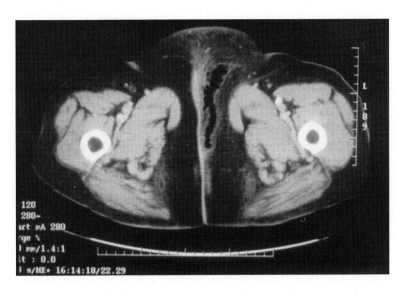

FIGURE 19.25 CT scan demonstrating necrotizing fasciitis of perineum.

TABLE 19.1 MICROBIOLOGY OF WOUND INFECTION AFTER CESAREAN DELIVERY

Isolate	Roberts et al. 1993 (N = 65)	Emmons et al. 1988 (N = 57)
Staphylococcus aureus	3 (5%)	16 (28%)
Staphylococcus epidermidis, coagulase-negative staphylococci	15 (23%)	19 (33%)
Facultative streptococci	14 (22%)	27 (47%)
Gram-negative rods	4 (6%)	16 (28%)
Anaerobes	7 (11%)	28 (49%)
Ureaplasma sp	29 (45%)	Not tested
Mycoplasma sp	10 (15%)	Not tested
No growth	18 (28%)	9 (11%)

Note: From Roberts S, Maccato M, Faro S, et al. The microbiology of post-cesarean wound morbidity. *Obstet Gynecol* 1993;81:383–386; Emmons SL, Krohn M, Jackson M, et al. Development of wound infections among women undergoing cesarean section. *Obstet Gynecol* 1988;72:559–564, with permission.

TABLE 19.2 DIAGNOSIS AND TREATMENT OF LIFE-THREATENING WOUND INFECTION

Condition	Signs/Symptoms	Organism	Treatment
Meleney gangrene (nonclostridial bacterial synergistic gangrene)	Slowly progressing pain, ulcer; ecchymosis erythema	Mixed	Broad-spectrum antibiotics, excision of skin, subcutaneous tissue
Necrotizing fascitis	Pain, edema, watery discharge—early; bullae—late	Mixed	Broad-spectrum antibiotics, excision of affected fascia with overlying skin, subcutaneous tissue
Clostridial myonecrosis (gas gangrene)	Pain; jaundice, crepitus; gas—late sign	*Clostridium perfringens*	Penicillin plus broad-spectrum coverage, excision of involved muscle (e.g., hysterectomy) or overlying tissues

BOX 19.1

Episiotomy Infections

Surgical exploration of episiotomy infections usually is indicated by:
- Extension beyond the labia
- Unilateral edema
- Systemic signs of toxicity or deterioration
- Failure of infection to resolve within 24–48 hours

20

PARASITIC DISEASE IN PREGNANCY

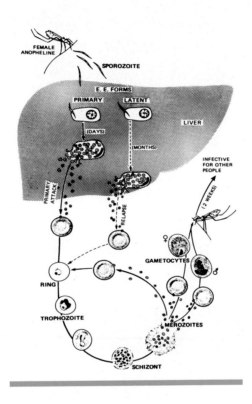

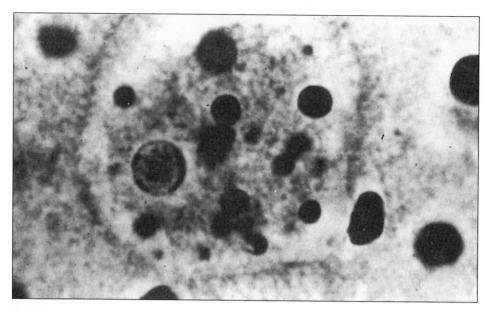

FIGURE 20.1 Trophozoites of *E. histolytica*. A delicate round nucleus is seen and the trophozoite contains ingested red blood cells. (From Ravdin JI, Petri WA Jr. Entamoeba histolytica (amebiasis). In: Mandel GL, Douglas RG, Bennett JE, eds. *Principles and practice of infectious diseases*. New York: John Wiley & Sons, 1990, with permission.)

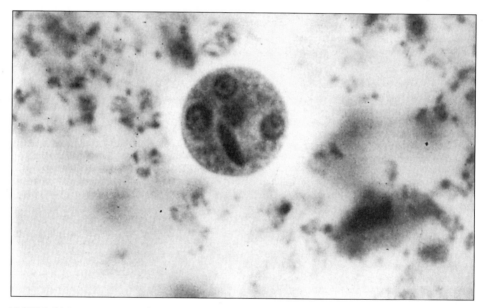

FIGURE 20.2 Mature cyst of *E. histolytica* with three of four nuclei seen. (From Ravdin JI, Petri WA Jr. Entamoeba histolytica (amebiasis). In: Mandel GL, Douglas RG, Bennett JE, eds. *Principles and practice of infectious diseases*. New York: John Wiley & Sons, 1990, with permission.)

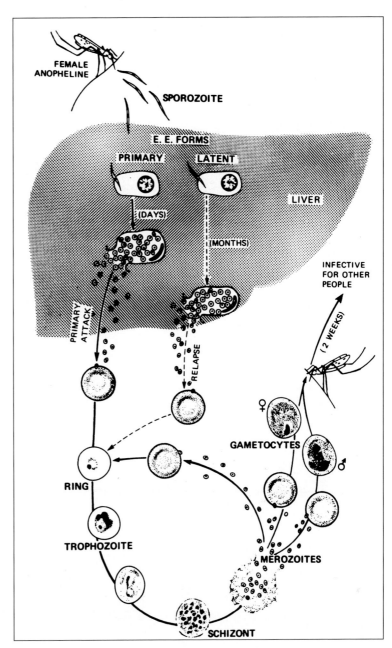

FIGURE 20.3 Life cycle of plasmodia in man. (From Wyler DJ, Miller LH. Plasmodium species. In: Mandel GL, Douglas RG, Bennett JE, eds. *Principles and practice of infectious diseases.* New York: John Wiley & Sons, 1979, with permission.)

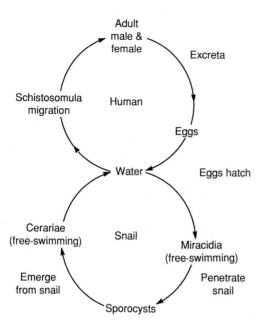

FIGURE 20.4 Life cycle of schistosomes. (From Miller LH. Plasmodium species. In: Mandell GL, Douglas RG, Bennett JE, eds. *Principles and practice of infectious disease.* New York: John Wiley & Sons, 1979, with permission.)

ANTIBIOTICS/ANTIVIRALS

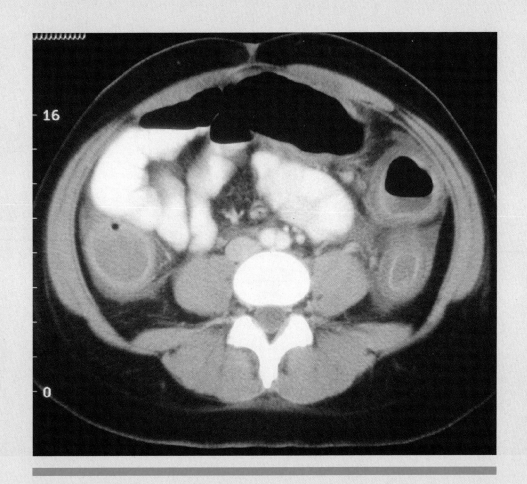

21

ANTIMICROBIAL AGENTS

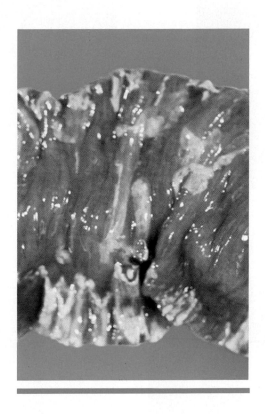

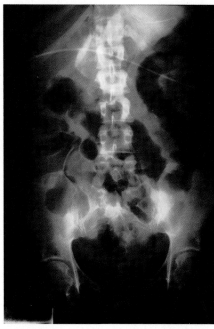

FIGURE 21.1 Radiograph showing a patient who had *Clostridium difficile*–associated diarrhea. The radiograph shows thickened bowel wall.

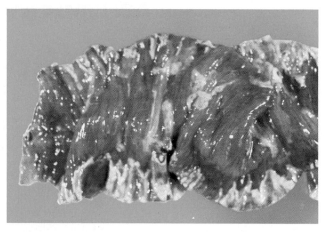

FIGURE 21.3 Gross appearance of bowel of patient with pseudomembranous enterocolitis.

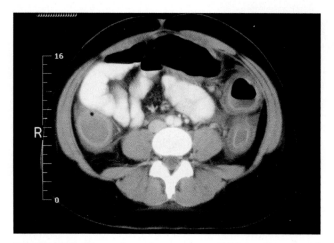

FIGURE 21.2 CT scan from the same case. Thickened bowel wall is noted clearly.

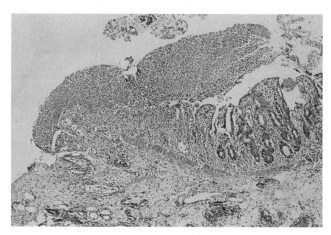

FIGURE 21.4 Microscopic appearance of bowel in case in Figure 21.3. Mucosa is normal in segments with abrupt changes to fibrinous plaques which replace the mucosa.

TABLE 21.1 POTENTIAL RISKS ASSOCIATED WITH ANTIMICROBIAL AGENTS IN PREGNANT AND LACTATING WOMEN

Use in Pregnancy, Agent	Maternal	Fetal	Excretion in Milk
	Type of Toxicity		
Contraindicated			
Chloramphenicol	Marrow aplasia	Gray syndrome	Yes
Tetracycline	Hepatotoxicity	Tooth discoloration and dysplasia	Yes
	Hemorrhagic pancreatitis	Inhibition of bone growth	Yes
	Renal failure		
Erythromycin estolate	Hepatotoxicity	None known	Yes
Quinolones (cinoxacin, norfloxacin, ofloxacin, ciprofloxacin)		Arthropathy in immature animals	Yes
Used with caution			
Aminoglycosides	Ototoxicity and nephrotoxicity	Eighth nerve toxicity	Yes
Clindamycin	Allergic reactions; pseudomembranous colitis	None known	Trace
Nitrofurantoin	Neuropathy	Hemolytis (glucose-6-phosbate dehydrogenase deficiency)	Trace
Metronidazole	Blood dyscrasia	Not known	Yes
Trimethoprim-sulfamethoxazole	Vasculitis	Folate antagonism	Yes
Sulfonamides	Allergic reactions	Kernicterus	Yes
Isoniazid	Hepatotoxicity	Possible neuropathy and seizures	Yes
Aztreonam	Allergic reactions	None known	Yes
Considered safe			
Penicillins	Allergic reactions	None known	Trace
Cephalosporins	Allergic reactions	None known	Trace
Erythromycin base	Allergic reactions	None known	Yes
Erythromycin ethinylsuccinate	Allergic reactions	None known	Yes
Spectinomycin	Allergic reactions	None known	Yes

Note: From Chow AW, Jewesson PJ. Pharmakinetics and safety of antimicrobial agents during pregnancy. *Rev Infect Dis* 1985;7:287–313, with permission.

TABLE 21.2 DOSING OF CIPROFLOXACIN AND OFLOXACIN[a]

Infection	Ciprofloxacin	Ofloxacin
Urinary tract		
Uncomplicated	250 mg q12h (3 d)	200 mg q12h (3 d)
Complicated	500 mg q12h (7 d)	200 mg q12h (7 d)
Infectious diarrhea	500 mg q12h	300 mg q12h
Lower respiratory, bone and joint, skin and skin structures		
Mild to moderate	500 mg q12h	400 mg q12h
Severe	750 mg q12h	
Acute uncomplicated gonorrhea	500 mg single dose	400 mg single dose
Chlamydia trachomatis cervicitus/urethritis	——	300 mg q12h (7 d)

[a] Oral and intravenous doses are same.

BOX 21.1
Classification of Cephalosporins

First generation
    Cefazolin (Ancef, Kefzol)
    Cephalexin (Keflex)
    Cefadroxil (Duricef, Ultracef)
Second generation
    Cefamandole (Mandol)
    Cefoxitin (Mefoxin)
    Cefotetan (Cefotan)
    Cefuroxime (Zinacef)
    Cefuroxime axetil (Ceftin)
    Cefaclor (Ceclor)
    Cefonicid (Monocid)
    Loracarbef (Lorabid)
    Cefprozil (Cefzil)
Third generation
    Cefotaxime (Claforan)
    Cefoperazone[a] (Cefobid)
    Ceftizoxime (Cefizox)
    Ceftriaxone (Rocephin)
    Ceftibuten (Cedax)
    Ceftazadime[a] (Fortaz)
    Cefixime (Suprax)
    Cefpodoxime proxetil (Vantin)
Fourth generation
    Cefepime (Maxipime)

---

[a] Third-generation cephalosporins with good antipseudomonas activity.

IMMUNIZATION

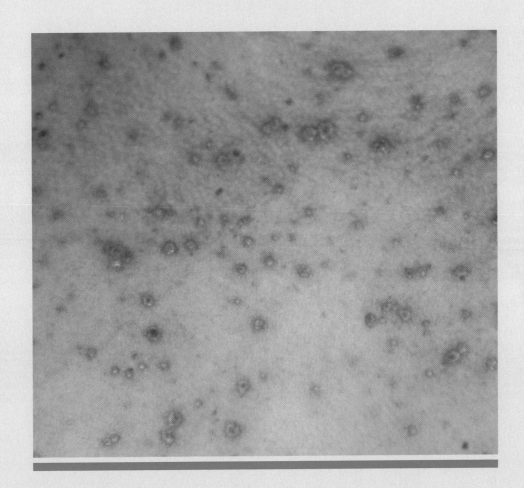

22

IMMUNIZATION

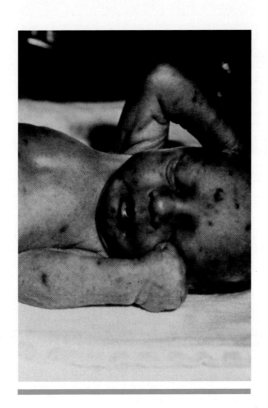

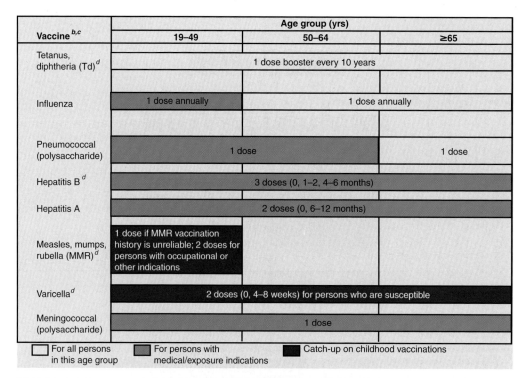

Vaccine [b,c]	Age group (yrs)		
	19–49	50–64	≥65
Tetanus, diphtheria (Td) [d]	1 dose booster every 10 years		
Influenza	1 dose annually	1 dose annually	
Pneumococcal (polysaccharide)	1 dose		1 dose
Hepatitis B [d]	3 doses (0, 1–2, 4–6 months)		
Hepatitis A	2 doses (0, 6–12 months)		
Measles, mumps, rubella (MMR) [d]	1 dose if MMR vaccination history is unreliable; 2 doses for persons with occupational or other indications		
Varicella [d]	2 doses (0, 4–8 weeks) for persons who are susceptible		
Meningococcal (polysaccharide)	1 dose		

☐ For all persons in this age group   ▨ For persons with medical/exposure indications   ■ Catch-up on childhood vaccinations

FIGURE 22.1 Recommended adult immunization schedule, by age group—United States, 2003–2004.[a] (From Centers for Disease Control and Prevention. *MMWR* 2003;52:965–69, with permission.)

[a] Approved by the Advisory Committee on Immunization Practices and accepted by the American College of Obstetricians and Gynecologists (ACOG) and the American Academy of Family Physicians (AAFP).

[b] This schedule indicates recommended age groups for routine administration of currently licensed vaccines for persons aged ≥19 years. Licensed combination vaccines may be used whenever any components of the combination are indicated and the vaccine's other components are not contraindicated.

[c] Additional information regarding these vaccines and contraindications for vaccination is available from the National Immunization Hotline (800-232-2522) or at the National Immunization Program's website (http://www.cdc.gov/nip).

[d] Covered by the Vaccine Injury Compensation Program (800-338-2382; http://.hrsa.gov/osp/vicp).

Medical condition	Vaccine						
	Tetanus-diphtheria (Td)	Influenza	Pneumo-coccal (polysac-charide)	Hepatitis B	Hepatitis A	Measles, mumps, rubella (MMR)	Varicella
Pregnancy		A					
Diabetes, heart disease, chronic pulmonary disease, and chronic liver disease, including chronic alcoholism		B	C		D		
Congenital immunodeficiency, leukemia, lymphoma, generalized malignancy, therapy with alkylating agents, antimetabolites, radiation, or large amounts of corticosteroids			E				F
Renal failure/end-stage renal disease and patients receiving hemodialysis or clotting factor concentrates			E	G			
Asplenia, including elective splenectomy and terminal complement-component deficiencies		H	E, I, J				
Human immunodeficiency virus (HIV) infection			E, K			L	

☐ For all persons in this group   ▓ For persons with medical/exposure indications   ■ Catch-up on childhood vaccinations   ▨ Contraindicated

FIGURE 22.2 Recommended adult immunization schedule, by medical condition—United States, 2003–2004. (From Centers for Disease Control and Prevention *MMWR* 2003;52:965–69, with permission.)

A. For women without chronic diseases/conditions, vaccinate if pregnancy will be at second or third trimester during influenza season. For women with chronic diseases/conditions, vaccinate at any time during the pregnancy.

B. Although chronic liver disease and alcoholism are not indicator conditions for influenza vaccination, administer 1 dose annually if the patient is aged >50 years, has other indications for influenza vaccine, or requests vaccination.

C. Asthma is an indicator condition for influenza but not for pneumococcal vaccination.

D. For all persons with chronic liver disease.

E. For persons aged <65 years, revaccinate once after ≥5 years have elapsed since initial vaccination.

F. Persons with impaired humoral but not cellular immunity may be vaccinated.

G. For hemodialysis patients use special formulation of vaccine (40 μg/mL) or two 1.0 mL 20 μg doses administered at one site. Vaccinate early in the course of renal disease. Assess antibody titers to hepatitis B surface antigen (anti-HBs) levels annually. Administer additional doses if anti-HBs levels decline to ≤10 mlU/mL.

H. No data have been reported specifically on risk for severe or complicated influenza infections among persons with asplenia. However, influenza is a risk factor for secondary bacterial infections that might cause severe disease in asplenics.

I. Administer meningococcal vaccine and consider *Haemophilus influenzae* type B vaccine.

J. In the event of elective splenectomy, vaccinate >2 weeks before surgery.

K. Vaccinate as close to diagnosis as possible when CD4 cell counts are highest.

L. Withhold MMR or other measles-containing vaccines from HIV-infected persons with evidence of severe immunosuppression.

INDEX

Note: Numbers with *t* indicate a table or boxed text; *f* indicates a figure or illustration.